"You need a di... bodily needs and the true purpose of foods. You need a diet and health plan you can stick to comfortably, with enjoyment, for the rest of your life."

Getting It Off, Keeping It Off is designed for those who are concerned about nutrition, health, and fitness. The GIO-KIO program — "God's diet plan" — is more than a plan for weight loss. By changing your perspective on food, this program will improve your self-confidence, increase your energy levels, and build your resistance to diseases. To inform and encourage you, Dr. Charles Salter includes actual menus and recipes, biblical teaching, and inspiring success stories. Because the GIO-KIO diet allows for personal food preferences, this is a plan you'll enjoy following. Adapt this sensible, effective, and easy-to-maintain program as your healthy, new life-style. You'll become the fit, attractive person you've always longed to be.

GETTING IT OFF KEEPING IT OFF

Charles A. Salter, Ph.D.

FLEMING H. REVELL COMPANY
OLD TAPPAN, NEW JERSEY

Library of Congress Cataloging-in-Publication Data

Salter, Charles A.
  Getting it off, keeping if off / by Charles A. Salter.
     p.   cm.
  ISBN 0-8007-5275-9
  1. Reducing. 2. Reducing—Religious aspects—Christianity.
I. Title.
RM222.2.S235 1988
613.2'5—dc19
                                                   87-36979
                                                        CIP

Copyright © 1988 by Charles A. Salter, Ph.D.
Published by Fleming H. Revell Company
Old Tappan, New Jersey 07675
Printed in the United States of America

TO
=

My children
Brian
Valerie
Carolyn

Thanks to
Mrs. Teresa McGraw, R.N.,
for her assistance in
collecting interview data

Contents

Section III:
Burning Up Calories

Section IV:
Changing Your Life

A word of caution: It is always advisable to consult with your own physician before beginning any sort of new diet. Let him or her know that this diet and health plan adheres to all the safety and health standards of the American Heart Association, the National Cancer Institute, the U.S. Department of Health and Human Services Dietary Guidelines, and the Human Nutrition Information Service of the U.S. Department of Agriculture.

However, the views, opinions, and findings in this book are those of the author and should not be construed as an official Department of the Army position, policy, or decision, unless so designated by other official documentation.

Preface

This book was written for a special person, you. You wouldn't have picked up this book if fat weren't on your mind. Maybe you are overweight or someone you love is fat. Maybe you have seen the needle on the bathroom scale move up farther over the years. Perhaps you are not all that fat right now but are worried about becoming overweight in the future.

If so, you are not alone. Nutrition experts tell us that 20 to 40 percent of all Americans are significantly overweight. And almost all adults could stand to lose a few pounds. Steven Gortmaker, my friend at Harvard University, has shown in his research that more and more children are becoming overweight. Nationwide, the problem is getting worse, not better.

I wasn't always concerned about fat; throughout high school I was the skinniest boy in my grade. I was always teased and subsequently pushed toward muscle-building programs and weight-adding diets. No matter what I did or how much I ate, I couldn't put on a pound. At seventeen I was nearly six feet tall and weighed all of 125 pounds. I was the original string bean!

But something happened as I entered my twenties and went to graduate school at the University of Pennsylvania. Although I didn't eat any more than before and didn't work any less, my metabolism slowed down, as does everyone's sooner or later. The weight started to ooze on like water from a leaky faucet. At first I was delighted to have some flesh on my bones. But the next thing you know, I had put on forty pounds in a couple of years. I was so fat that everyone started teasing me for that!

Talk about injustices! I went from ridicule for being too skinny to jeers for being too fat. There was never an in-between time when people thought I looked just right. Never!

I read all kinds of diet books and watched the diet experts on TV. I dabbled in different diets and lost a few pounds here and there. For a while. Then the weight came back on, plus a little extra.

It became clear I wasn't the only one concerned about fat. As a college psychology professor I noted that most teenagers and young adults are concerned about their bodily fat and appearance. Later, through my nationally syndicated column, I became more aware that practically everyone is concerned about their weight and health.

All the fad diets seemed to make little sense; I wanted the real answers. So I went to Harvard University and spent two years taking every nutrition course I could. I even earned my master of science degree in nutrition there.

I soon realized the most amazing thing: The latest scientific findings were coming closer and closer to saying what the Bible had already said about diet and health thousands of years ago! In between the original Bible truths and the cutting edge of today's science were the trendy diets and hokey stuff you see in the media. But the best of science was cutting through the garbage and catching up to where the Bible had been all along.

Talk about good news! I knew this story had to be told and I knew you would want to know. What follows is the result of my years of study and research into both science and the Bible.

The message is wonderful:

You *can* gain control over your fat problem.

You *can* lose your extra weight. And keep it off.

You *can* still enjoy food and eat all the things you like.

You *can* look and feel better, starting from the first day.

The scientific way, the Bible way, has worked for me, and it can work for you. I lost my unwanted fat, put on a few pounds of muscle, strengthened my heart and lungs, and increased my endurance.

You don't have to mope around so hungry that you're depressed and irritable all the time. I know you're afraid of that. In my fad diet days I wrestled with intense hunger and know how you feel. Starving yourself is not the answer and you won't find that here.

This is not just a diet. The Getting It Off, Keeping It Off (GIO-KIO) plan is a *complete* health plan. You'll lose weight, but you'll also look and feel healthier. You'll have more energy, more vigor, and more resistance to stress and disease. So read on and start becoming in real life the thin, attractive, healthy person you've always wanted to be. Don't wait a moment longer!

STARTING TODAY
YOU
WILL GAIN CONTROL
OVER YOUR WEIGHT
PROBLEM

Section I

Seeing Where You Stand Now

1

Rich Food, Poor Body

Could you increase your life span by another five to twenty years if you lost excess weight and changed to a healthier diet? Would you be fitter, more robust, and happier with a better diet?

My professors in nutrition at Harvard University's School of Public Health have investigated this issue. The Framingham Heart Study, under the direction of William Castelli, has followed over five thousand men and women for more than three decades and kept records on their diets, activities, health, and longevity. One finding suggests that improving the diet remarkably reduces the risks of heart disease. Even a little dietary improvement can have some beneficial effects.

I'm sure the prophet Daniel would have agreed with this conclusion that a better diet might save your life and improve your health and appearance.

Daniel's Ten-Day Diet Challenge

How would you feel if your homeland were attacked by a foreign army, you were taken captive, and, scared to death, you got sent not to the salt mines but to the royal court of the enemy leader? You're a captive, but at least you have it better than any of your countrymen. Would you be willing to complain about the food, or would you thank your lucky stars that you weren't stuck doing slave labor?

The Book of Daniel in the Bible describes just such a scenario, beginning around the year 605 B.C. As a young man the prophet Daniel and his friends Shadrach, Meshach, and Abednego were captured by the Babylonians, who had marched on Jerusalem to put down the rebellion there. Many of the Hebrew captives no doubt were forced into abject slavery. But something about Daniel and his friends—their obvious talent and health, perhaps—caught the eye of one of the Babylonian officers. Daniel and his friends were selected to serve at a high level in the royal court of King Nebuchadnezzar. They were to be trained for three years and receive rich food and wine from the king's own table.

This was considered a great honor, of course. Daniel wasn't going to have to eat slop and dig ditches. He would be treated like a prince, probably better than any of the other captured Hebrews.

But God told Daniel to avoid the king's rich food and wine. It wasn't healthy. What kind of menu did the king serve, anyway?

The Bible doesn't say, but we know from independent historical sources that the Babylonian diet included butter, cheese, fish, mutton, beef, pork, poultry, honey, and palm sugar.[1] It emphasized beer and various kinds of wine. The Babylonians especially prized animal fat, particularly fat pork. Ancient letters mention oxen that were made so fat prior to butchering they couldn't even stand up!

The king's diet was much too rich in alcohol, grease, animal fats, cholesterol, and sugar. If that sounds familiar, you're right: The average American diet in this century has been catching up to the Babylonian luxury diet.

Anyway, Daniel decided that he wouldn't defile himself with the king's extravagant food. He asked the chief eunuch to let him avoid this rich diet. The chief eunuch was terrified at the thought. Like many people today, he thought that such a rich diet was actually good for you. What could be better than gorging on the finest food in the land? He feared that Daniel and his friends would start to waste away on any lesser diet. The king would notice their poor physical condition, blame the chief eunuch for not fulfilling his duty, and probably have him beheaded.

But God made the chief eunuch favorably disposed toward Daniel. The man agreed to Daniel's request for a ten-day trial. He would let Daniel and his friends eat their "inferior" diet for ten days and then see the result. He probably figured that they couldn't get too sickly in just ten days. They would start to look a little weaker, he guessed, and then he would prove to Daniel that this other diet was foolish. Daniel would certainly want to go back to the "superior" Babylonian diet.

What kind of diet did Daniel propose? No fat, sugar, and alcohol. He wanted just vegetables and water. (That was all for the first ten days, although he added more things later, as we'll see.)

We have here the first known test of two different diet plans. The challenge Daniel issued sounds much like many modern diet plans today: "Try this new diet and lose up to ten pounds a week." The difference is that God inspired Daniel's diet plan.

At the end of the ten-day trial, Daniel and his friends looked healthier and better nourished than any of the young men their age who were eating the Babylonian diet. The chief eunuch was amazed! He had the guard take away their rich food and wine (Daniel 1).

Does this diet comparison mean we should all become vegetarians? No, of course not. Part of Daniel's motivation was simply his desire to stick true to Jewish dietary laws, which generally do not apply to Christians today. The Bible clearly states elsewhere that God provides all kinds of meat as well as plant products for human food (Mark 7:19; Romans 14:14). Furthermore, we know from Daniel 10:3 that Daniel also ate meat and drank wine later when he had more freedom.

Probably the reason Daniel chose only vegetables and water in those ten days is that those were the only items on that particular menu that seemed suitable. In other words, the guard delivered to Daniel the regular rich diet and Daniel selected and ate only the healthiest items from that sumptuous spread. Then the guard later had to take away the fatty and sweet items that Daniel left behind. But once Daniel rose to power in the Babylonian kingdom, he was able to have his own cooks prepare healthier meals of vegetables and meat and so on.

The point is not to throw away your meat and eat only vegetables. Rather, you should eat a balanced diet of vegetables and other things, properly selected and prepared. What God told Daniel some twenty-five centuries ago has finally been documented by modern nutritional science: Too much rich food and wine is bad for your physical health, mental health, and appearance.

The Miraculous Effects of Vegetables

It was not until the 1980s that nutritionists documented the almost miraculous effect of vegetables on the body. Frank Sacks, an assistant professor of medicine at Brigham and Women's Hospital in Boston and a lecturer in nutrition at Harvard, has investigated the effects of diet on blood pressure. To understand his findings, you need to realize that high blood pressure is bad; it's unhealthy. A lower blood pressure is usually a good sign of improved health. Dr. Sacks cites a number of scientific studies that indicate a high vegetable diet significantly lowers blood pressure.

Dr. Sacks and his colleagues discovered that vegetarians typically have lower blood pressure than meat-eating people of the same age and sex.[2] Another study showed that normal meat eaters who went on a vegetarian diet for a few weeks had a significant drop in blood pressure.[3] However, Sacks also studied a group of strict vegetarians who were asked to add meat to their diets for a few weeks.[4] Their overall blood pressure did not shoot up dramatically. Dr. Sacks concluded that cutting out meat products does not lower blood pressure. It is adding vegetables that helps. So you don't have to become a vegetarian to have a healthy diet. You just need to add more vegetables to whatever diet you already have.

Bruce Ames of the department of biochemistry at the University of California at Berkeley has focused his research on the effect of vegetables on cancer. Some of his findings are no less than astounding.[5]

- Whole-grain cereals, vegetable oils, and peanuts contain vitamin E, which helps protect the body against cancer and other illnesses.
- Carrots and other yellow and green vegetables contain carotenoids, which help prevent cancer, even in those who smoke.
- Citrus fruits, potatoes, tomatoes, and green leafy vegetables contain vitamin C, which helps the body resist cancers, particularly those related to ultraviolet radiation (of the sun).
- Whole grains also contain selenium (as do certain vegetables grown in selenium-containing soil). This mineral protects against cancer, heart disease, and the poisonous effects of other chemicals.

Your mother was right all along (though perhaps she didn't know exactly why) when she said, "Eat your vegetables, they're good for you!"

Poor Diet Can Kill

A poor diet not only makes you look and feel worse, it saps your inner strength and vitality. It makes you fall prey to various diseases and it can actually kill you.

The National Center for Health Statistics released the following figures on the leading causes of death in the United States in 1984.[6] The causes of death are listed in order of frequency and I have added some possible dietary contributors to these problems.

Leading Causes of Death

Rank	Cause	Death Rate Per 100,000	Dietary Contributions
1	Cancer	791.3	High fat, low fiber
2	Cardiovascular disease	409.2	Excess animal fats
3	Accidents	39.9	Excess alcohol
4	Chronic lung disease	29.6	Malnutrition; smoking
5	Influenza and pneumonia	24.7	Malnutrition
6	Diabetes mellitus	15.1	Excess sugar
7	Suicide	11.8	Depression may be related to poor diet
8	Cirrhosis of liver	11.3	Excess alcohol

In all these eight leading causes of death, diet may play some role. In some cases diet is the most important factor. For example, excess animal fat seems to be the main determinant of atherosclerosis or clogged arteries, a major type of cardiovascular disease. The fats actually form more and more deposits inside the arteries, gradually closing the opening and reducing the flow of blood, thus inducing heart attacks and strokes. As the following chart shows, as cholesterol (from animal fats in the diet) increases in the blood, so does the incidence of coronary heart disease.[7]

These numbers might make more sense with an example. Your doctor can order a blood test for you that will reveal the amount of cholesterol in your blood. A person with a reading of 240, for instance, has about twice the chance of developing heart disease as a person with 220 (the risk of 47 per thousand is about twice that of 22). In general, the lower your blood cholesterol, the better.

Blood Cholesterol (mg per 100 ml)	Coronary Heart Disease (cases per 1000)
Less than 204	9
205–234	22
235–264	47
265–294	59
Over 295	116

Note: These data are rounded figures for a six-year period of risk for men from thirty to forty-nine years of age. The data vary somewhat for men of other ages and for women.

Let me also give a personal example. I knew years ago that a cholesterol reading over about 220, if maintained for years, can spell real danger to your heart. Some experts now think a reading above 200 is too risky. Before taking Daniel's ten-day diet challenge, my own reading was about 198, right around 200. It was borderline healthy because I was already using exercise and a reduced-fat diet. But a few weeks after I followed the even healthier plan which is outlined in this book, my reading dropped by 33 points to 165!

If you are concerned about your own cholesterol standing, ask your doctor to tell you the results of your last blood test. If it's been a while since you had one, ask for another or, better yet, a complete physical exam.

Similarly, a high-fat and low-fiber diet can increase the risk of some cancers. Too much sugar in the diet can help cause or worsen diabetes in those who are susceptible. Such persons cannot produce enough insulin to handle the excess sugar, or their bodies can't use insulin in the normal way to do so.

For other causes of death a dietary role is possible, but less certain. Being overweight and eating the wrong kinds of food can help cause or increase depression. This may in turn lead to suicide, but there are obviously other factors involved.

Being Overweight Can Kill

Besides eating the wrong kinds of food, eating the wrong amounts can kill you. You could eat a diet balanced for all the different nutrients but eat too much. Whenever you eat more calories than your body uses, the extra is converted into fat. If you keep eating more than you use day after day, you'll keep putting on more and more fat.

Obesity has been linked to the following:[8]

- Heart problems
- Arthritis
- Gallbladder problems, including gallstones
- Uterine, bile-duct, and breast cancer in women
- Colon, rectal, and prostate cancer in men

In general the fatter you are, the greater your risk of death from one of these or related causes. As the percentage of your body weight goes up above normal, so does your chance of dying at a given age. In the following table the average death rate is set at 100:[9]

Percent of Ideal Body Weight	Death Rate
100	100
130	135
160	210

These particular data hold for men fifteen to thirty-nine years old. If a man is at the ideal weight (e.g., 150 pounds) for his height and age, his chances of death are normal. But if he is at 130 percent of his ideal body weight, that is, 30 percent overweight (e.g., 150 + 45 = 195 lb.), his chances of death at that age go up by an additional 35 percent. That is, his death rate is 135 rather than 100. If he is 60 percent overweight (e.g., 150 + 90 = 240 lb.), his risk of death more than doubles (210 versus 100). In general the more overweight, the greater the overall chances of death from all causes combined.

For women, the impact of obesity on death rates is somewhat lower than for men, but still serious.

So much for the bad news. The good news is that if you lose the extra weight, your chances of death due to obesity decline gradually back toward normal. Your chances of getting these various diseases also decline. And if you've already developed one of them, its severity can be markedly reduced by a healthy diet. For example, adult-onset diabetes can now be controlled, usually by diet and exercise alone.[10]

God's Plan

Right now you are probably in one of three categories:

1. Your current weight is okay, but you want to keep it that way and maximize your chances for a lifetime of good health.
2. You are slightly overweight and want to lose a few pounds. You want to have more energy and feel better.
3. You are clearly overweight (at least 20 percent) and want to lose many pounds. You are concerned about your physical image and how people look at you. You want to be more accepted by others and more able to like yourself. You are concerned that excess fat can cut years off your life, and reduce the amount of life in your years.

Whichever category you are in, I urge you to accept Daniel's ten-day diet challenge. Try this approach for just ten days and see if you don't look and feel better, starting almost immediately.

You've probably spent a lifetime—twenty or forty or sixty years—building bad eating habits. You've gotten stuck in the overeater's lane in our society, or you've tried weird, fashionable, or trendy diets that weaken you and make you sick. Is ten days too much time to spend proving to yourself once and for all that you can take charge of enriching your life? I promise you this: *In less than even one day you will start to look and feel better.*

After you've spent ten days breaking old habits and purifying your system, you'll be in a position to build new habits. It won't just be veggies and water—remember, even Daniel didn't stick with that all his life. With the GIO-KIO (Getting It Off, Keeping It Off) plan, you'll learn how to eat, for the first time in your life, a truly balanced diet that matches the requirements of your body, as God designed it, with the nature of foods, as God made them.

With this approach to weight control and health, you will do the following:

- Enjoy all the foods that God has richly bestowed on us
- Lose unneeded and unsightly pounds of fat
- Get your weight down and keep it down *permanently*
- Reduce your chances of death from obesity-related causes and poor diet
- Improve your appearance
- Improve your self-confidence and social appeal
- Increase your muscle strength and vigor
- Improve your mental and physical ability to work and play, to serve God
- Better conform your eating attitudes and habits to God's plan, thus improving your spiritual life
- Avoid or break free from harmful food addictions and compulsions, or from dangerous eating disorders like anorexia and bulimia

You'll see many diet books on the shelves today that promise to help you control weight. The best of them, though incomplete, are just beginning to catch up to God's plan written in the Bible thousands of years ago! Why settle for less when you can get the straight facts from the original source, from the One who created both food and the human body?

TOO MUCH
RICH FOOD
MAKES A
POOR BODY

2

Do You Need to Lose Weight?

Not everyone needs to lose weight. If you don't, then you might want to skip this chapter. The GIO-KIO plan is a complete health program that covers more than losing pounds. So if your weight is fine as is, go ahead to chapter 3.

What do we mean by being overweight? Some people think that if you are not gaunt, with tight skin and no sign of fat anywhere, you are overweight. But that image of the ultrathin, scrawny model who is always starving herself is a distortion of the real meaning of normal weight. Some body fat is completely normal. In fact, if you literally got rid of all your body fat, you would die.

By overweight I *don't* mean that you weigh just a couple of pounds over what you'd like to weigh, or that you can feel a little soft fat on your arm or tummy. If that's your only fat problem, you don't have a fat problem! By overweight I mean that you weigh at least 20 percent more than you should for your sex, height, and body build (an upcoming table will show what your ideal body weight should be). For example, if you should weigh 130 pounds but really weigh 156 or more (20 percent of 130 = 26; 130 + 26 = 156), you probably are overweight and could afford to lose some of that extra fat.

Causes of Being Overweight

Heredity

The genes you inherited from your parents have a lot to do with your overall size, basic body frame, and how easily you convert calories into fat. Two people could eat exactly the same diet every day, spend the same amount of calories on work and exercise every day, and yet one could stay thin and the other could put on fat.

The naturally thin person burns up more calories in metabolic processes. But the sad truth for many overweight people is that their bodies tend to store rather than burn excess calories. It doesn't seem fair, does it? Some people start off life slim, but as their metabolic rate declines with age, they start putting on weight. If you fit into that category, take heart, for we will see later a marvelous way you can turn up your metabolic furnace and burn more of those extra calories than you ever have before.

Here are some signs that you might be in this category:

- One or both of your parents is overweight, in spite of normal eating
- Several of your other relatives are overweight, in spite of normal eating
- You seem to put on weight even when eating no more than much thinner people

If even one of these signs holds true for you, you may fit into this category.

For instance, Sara complained to me about her difficulty in losing weight. She describes herself as an intelligent, grossly overweight nurse who enjoys eating and becomes depressed when dieting. She is thirty-nine years old, divorced, and active in her church. Her former approach to weight control was to reduce the variety of foods she ate (not a good idea!) and to eat less. But she ate so little at certain times that she suffered muscle cramps, nausea, and a kind of mental fogginess. This interfered with her job performance and daily happiness. No wonder she got depressed when dieting! After all that suffering, she would eventually stop dieting and gain back all the lost weight anyhow.

Sara is one of the poor unfortunates who has inherited fat genes from fat parents. Her approach to controlling her weight, with seesaw extremes, just made the problem worse.

Glands and Hormones

There is a complicated hormonal interaction that helps to control the rate of metabolism and calorie use. Sometimes that system gets out of balance and produces overweight. An underactive thyroid or pituitary gland, for example, can tend to make you fat. That's fairly rare, but it does happen.

I had a friend who came from a fairly thin family in which everyone had reasonably good eating habits. My friend was quite thin until he turned about eleven or twelve. Then, practically overnight, he turned into a butterball, to everyone's amazement. This kind of sudden weight gain in the absence of obvious life-style changes made his family suspicious. They took him to the doctor, who soon discovered a thyroid deficiency. Regular medications quickly restored his hormonal balance, and the extra fat vanished as swiftly as it had appeared. (By the way, if you are fat despite having a normal hormone balance, you don't want to mess with your hormone system to try and lose weight artificially. That would create another kind of potentially serious hormone imbalance.)

The following is a key sign that a glandular hormone change might be responsible for your problem: if it developed rather suddenly—you were normal weight before that, and suddenly began to balloon out—but without any other obvious changes in diet or life-style. A hormone problem is not indicated if you gained weight suddenly because of divorce, depression, or other obvious problem and then began to overeat like crazy. If you have any doubt about your hormone status, have your physician give you a thorough checkup.

Inactivity

Probably the most common reason for creeping overweight in our society is simple inactivity. We may actually eat a reasonable amount for our body type and nutritional needs, but we are not using our bodies nearly as much as we should, far less than most humans have for the last several centuries. That is, we are consuming a reasonable number of calories, but we simply aren't burning as many as we should.

I once had a neighbor who wouldn't even walk the sixty feet from her front door to the mailbox every morning. There was nothing wrong with her legs, but she preferred to walk the ten feet from her back door to the car. Then she would drive to the front of her own house, get the mail, and drive back around to the garage again. I never once, in several years, saw this woman engage in any other kind of exercise, either.

A study conducted at the New England Medical Center and Harvard University discovered that the more children watch TV, the more likely they are to become obese.[1] Inactivity in front of the television uses few calories, and it takes away the normal play time that children could be spending on far more vigorous activities.

If you never or rarely exercise, you probably fit into this category. We'll discuss exercise more in chapter 11. Here are some possible signs that you are physically out of shape:

- Simple physical exertions (like carrying in the groceries) that you used to do with ease now seem much too difficult
- You huff and puff or feel the strain with even a little bit of exertion, as when climbing one flight of stairs
- Your heart seems to pound with any form of physical effort

If you are out of shape, start thinking about getting back to a more active life-style. If you have any doubt about what shape you're in, check with your doctor. He or she can give you stress tests and other heart tests to make sure that exercise is safe for you.

Eating for the Wrong Reasons

The right reason to eat is that you are hungry. God built the hunger start-and-stop signals into the body to help regulate your weight at normal levels and get the energy and nutrition you need to stay healthy. If you ate at the right speed, ate the right foods, ate only when you were hungry, and *stopped eating when you were no longer hungry*, you would have no trouble reaching and maintaining a reasonable weight.

Most people run into problems because they eat for the following wrong reasons, when they are not even hungry:

- You eat more than you want to please others or to meet some image of yourself (e.g., someone who always "cleans his plate").
- You eat out of habit, as when watching sports or TV.
- You eat to make yourself feel better when you are blue or feeling rejected or upset.

Habitual eating when you are not hungry immediately adds more calories than you can deal with, which are quickly turned into fat. Worse, over the long run habitual eating makes you less sensitive to your hunger start-and-stop signals so that you lose the ability of this natural system to regulate your weight properly. People who habitually overeat no longer realize when their body is trying to tell them to *stop* eating, as people stuck on fad diets often lose the ability to realize when their bodies are trying to tell them to *start* eating. If you have this problem, begin tuning in more to your body's natural hunger start-and-stop signals.

Self-Indulgence

Being overweight is sometimes (but certainly not always) linked with self-indulgence and self-absorption. At the extreme, overweight may ultimately be coupled with even corruption and wickedness.

Obesity in the Bible.   Judges 3 describes an obese man, Eglon, king of Moab. He was one of the evil rulers used by God to punish the Israelites when they turned away from Him. Eglon conquered the Israelites and kept them as subjects for eighteen years. He probably spent a lot of time feasting and lounging around like the Babylonians, who were discussed in the last chapter. Eglon was corrupt and enjoyed lording it over his subjects. He relished his power over the Israelites, exacting tribute from them to fill his royal treasury.

Then God sent Ehud to deliver Israel from this bondage. Ehud was chosen to present the tribute to Eglon, but he brought more than just money—he carried a hidden eighteen-inch sword. Drawing the king aside privately, he lunged the weapon right into his swollen belly. "And the hilt also went in after the blade, and the fat closed over the blade, for he did not draw the sword out of his belly . . . " (Judges 3:22).

This guy was enormous! Far from having a trim thirty-two- or thirty-four-inch waist, I estimate he would have had at least a sixty to accommodate an eighteen-inch sword in this way. Notice how this rampant obesity was associated with unchecked corruption and evil. Here was a man who had no control over his appetite for food, conquest, and tribute.

In the New Testament we have several cases of wealthy people who were absorbed with themselves and gave themselves over to sumptuous feasting. The Bible doesn't explicitly say that they were obese, but we can probably assume they were overweight from lounging around and overeating. We have the selfish rich man who wouldn't share even the crumbs from his sumptuous table with the beggar Lazarus (Luke 16:19–31). There was the prosperous farmer who decided to tear down his old barns, build larger ones, and then take life easy, eat, drink, and be merry (Luke 12:16–21). As you recall, both of these greedy men were sorely punished.

Obesity in history. Do you remember King Henry VIII of England? He had no control over his appetite for food, women, or power. He feasted himself into enormous obesity. To marry new wives, he practiced every kind of treachery to get rid of his old ones. If he couldn't divorce these poor women, he had them beheaded. Like Henry, many kings, emperors, shahs, sultans, and other selfish leaders over the centuries have been overweight due to indulgence. Their loss of self-control revealed itself in other areas besides food such as drinking, sex, and gambling.

Historically, it was only wealthy and powerful people who were able to deliberately overeat and laze around to the point of obesity. In most modern, advanced, democratic societies, all but the poorest citizens are able to practice gluttony if they so choose. But it isn't considered one of the seven deadly sins for nothing! Gluttony *kills*.

This is not to say that self-indulgence is the only cause of being fat. I certainly do not mean to imply that all overweight people are wicked or selfish! As I pointed out, there are many quite innocent causes of being overweight. A person born with fat genes, for instance, has no say in the matter. (However, with effort he can still overcome this genetic handicap to a large extent.)

Testing Yourself for Overweight

You probably already know whether or not you are overweight. If you are not sure, take one or more of these tests.

- Pinch yourself. The well-known saying if you can pinch an inch you have fat to lose is based on a valid truth. The amount of fat attached to your skin is a good measure of the total fat in your body. The back of your upper arm, rather than the belly, is the best place to check. If you are unsure about the result, your doctor can use this same fatfold test with finely measured calipers to be sure.
- Use a tape measure. Compare your chest (not bust) size in inches to your waist size. Ideally, the waist size should be less. If it's not, your stomach probably has too much fat.
- Look at yourself in the mirror. If you see extra folds of flesh hanging from a double chin, stomach, or hips, you

have excess fat. This mirror test, however, is not always reliable. Some anorexics starve themselves into looking like skeletons and yet think they still see fat. (Some fat is not only good for you, it is absolutely essential to sustain life. Being *too* thin is just as dangerous as being too fat).

• Look at your ideal body weight in the following height/weight table. See if your actual body weight is significantly higher than that. If it is 20 percent or more in excess of that ideal figure, you are overweight by definition.

To use this chart, look under the correct column for your sex.[2] Look for the line that gives your height without shoes. If you have a small body frame, look in the low-weight column. If you have a large, big-boned frame, look in the high-weight column. The majority of people have an average frame and can use the average column. Measure your weight with no clothing on and see how you compare. If you are just a couple of pounds above these standard figures, don't worry. But if you are starting to edge toward the next higher category, you may be in need of the GIO-KIO plan for weight control.

Turn now to Appendix B for your personalized Weight Loss Chart. Write down your current weight. Consider prayerfully what your goal weight should be in light of the weight table or the other tests. Now commit yourself in prayer to reaching this goal.

How You Stack Up

| Height (without shoes) | Weight (without clothing) | | |
	Low	Average	High
Men	Pounds	Pounds	Pounds
5 feet 3 inches	118	129	141
5 feet 4 inches	122	133	145
5 feet 5 inches	126	137	149
5 feet 6 inches	130	142	155
5 feet 7 inches	134	147	161

| Height (without shoes) | Weight (without clothing) | | |
	Low	Average	High
Men	Pounds	Pounds	Pounds
5 feet 8 inches	139	151	166
5 feet 9 inches	143	155	170
5 feet 10 inches	147	159	174
5 feet 11 inches	150	163	178
6 feet	154	167	183
6 feet 1 inch	158	171	188
6 feet 2 inches	162	175	192
6 feet 3 inches	165	178	195
Women			
5 feet	100	109	118
5 feet 1 inch	104	112	121
5 feet 2 inches	107	115	125
5 feet 3 inches	110	118	128
5 feet 4 inches	113	122	132
5 feet 5 inches	116	125	135
5 feet 6 inches	120	129	139
5 feet 7 inches	123	132	142
5 feet 8 inches	126	136	146
5 feet 9 inches	130	140	151
5 feet 10 inches	133	144	156
5 feet 11 inches	137	148	161
6 feet	141	152	166

Source: L. Page and L. J. Fincher, Food and Your Weight, Home
and Garden Bulletin no. 74 (Washington, D. C.: U. S. Government
Printing Office, 1967), p. 2.

Success Can Be Yours

Other than at special times of fasting, Christ enjoyed food.
The Bible records Jesus eating and drinking at many festivals,
parties, and banquets. But He also worked and exercised hard.

He kept His body in shape and took good care of it. You can't imagine Him being at all fat.

Christians are called to follow His example (1 Peter 2:21). And 2 Corinthians 3:18 adds, "And we all, with unveiled face, beholding the glory of the Lord, are being changed into his likeness from one degree of glory to another; for this comes from the Lord, who is the Spirit." In other words, the stronger we grow in the faith, the more we let the Spirit fill our lives, the more like Jesus we become.

Isn't it remarkable that for thousands of years being fat was considered a sign of health, wealth, and prosperity? It has only been in recent times that doctors have proven the risks of being overweight. But the Bible all along took a dim view of extravagant self-indulgence that leads to obesity. Once again we see modern science finally beginning to catch up to some of the truths long waiting for us in the Bible.

And putting them into practice can make a real difference in our lives.

Sally is a lovely young woman about five feet, five inches tall. But she ballooned out to 180 pounds in the first few years of her marriage. She has a large frame, but she was still about forty-five pounds overweight. Then she became a Christian. She soon realized the need to get her life in order, including her diet. Using the willpower that God gave her, she got her weight down to around 134 pounds. She has kept it there for many years now. She sings in the church choir and leads the children's choir. And few would ever guess that she was not always the svelte beauty she is now.

If this is the kind of change you need in your life, take heart: With God's help, you can do it, too!

YOU CAN
TAKE OFF
EXCESS WEIGHT
AND
KEEP IT OFF

3

Do You Need to Change Your Diet?

If you want to lose weight, you already know you need to change your diet. But even if you are one of the fortunate few with a normal weight, you may still need to change your diet for other health reasons. A person may never gain an ounce her entire lifetime, yet still turn fatter and fatter. How? This can happen if she lets the strong bone and muscle waste away and be replaced by fat. If body fat is not your problem, you may just need a healthier diet to keep your body strong and better able to resist disease.

Protect Your Body

The old saying "You are what you eat" is true. Your body processes whatever you eat, good or bad. Eating nothing but junk is like trying to build a house out of straw and sand. You may be able to produce a shelter, but it's not strong, and it doesn't last long.

If you eat a balanced, healthy diet, you are building a mansion from the finest brick and stone. Your bodily structure will be more sturdy and elegant and it will last longer and look better.

41

What kind of "house" have you been building for yourself so far in your life? We should remember that our bodies are temples of the Holy Spirit, and that we should honor God in our bodies (1 Corinthians 6:19–20). That's a scary thought, isn't it? It challenges us to take care of ourselves in many ways, including diet and health care.

Protect Your Self-Image

If we don't respect our own bodies, we begin to lose respect for ourselves as persons.

Paul, a thirty-three-year-old man, is married, works as a bank executive, and is an active volunteer worker in the community. He once weighed 250 pounds and was ashamed of his weight, as were his children. He said then that he was bored, depressed, and not happy with himself: "I would like to lose this weight. I feel if I liked myself better I could stick with a diet, but it is a vicious circle. The fat is the problem. I need to find the starting point." Isn't it sad that his weight was affecting his self-image and happiness? Once he got started on a serious diet, he was able to lose thirty pounds. He needs to lose still more, and I believe with God's help he can do it.

Lucy, fifty-two years old, tells a similar story at first. She is married and works as a receptionist. She says, "I want to lose weight but eat when unhappy or frustrated. Fad diets are not good. I'm still trying to find the secret and will try again."

Lucy illustrates again that vicious circle. Sometimes our fat makes us unhappy, so we eat to make ourselves feel better. But the overeating just makes us fatter and so on and so on.

But Lucy goes on to tell that the support of friends and family finally helped her overcome her lack of willpower. In just three months, she lost twenty pounds, declining from 170 to 150. Now she says, "Desire and willpower are the secrets of dieting success."

Lucy was able to break out of that vicious circle of fat-depression-overeating. With the help of others she was able to regain enough self-respect to assert control over her life. Now she can cope with unhappiness and frustration without running to the refrigerator for an extra slice of cheesecake or a bowl of ice cream.

Be a Soldier of God

As a researcher for the Department of Defense, I have worked with all branches of the military to help test and implement new foods and food-service systems. When developing a new military ration system, we try out sample batches of a variety of new menus. We keep only those the troops say they like. If there is something that most people don't like, we discard it from the system.

This leaves us with high-preference items but not a very balanced diet. We then add extra nutrients, even to items like crackers and chocolate, so that the troops can get enough of the right vitamins and minerals.

Our troops almost always eat a fairly balanced diet, whether they realize it or not. And they exercise well and practice self-discipline. This change in life-style *always* results in a marked difference in physique, personality, and self-confidence.

Most people coming into the military from homes with uncontrolled diets start off with lots of flab and little energy. But under the more regimented diet and exercise of basic training, in a few weeks they emerge leaner, fitter, and healthier than ever before.

Could it be that we are called to be soldiers of Christ (2 Timothy 2:3) in part for the same reason? Doesn't being more fit and trim help us better take our places in the Lord's army? And won't our Commanding Officer help us to get into shape if we ask Him?

You wouldn't have thought of my friend Mary as a soldier if you saw her before she started God's diet plan. She was forty-five, married, a secretary, and a volunteer worker for a cancer society. Her 150 pounds were far too much for her tiny frame to carry. But then like a good soldier she got, as she calls it, "motivation, determination, self-discipline." On her diet she had a good feeling of physical energy and mental clarity, just the opposite of what most people feel on fad diets. And she relished the positive comments she received as the weight melted off and she slimmed down to 119 pounds. She had to buy new clothing in smaller sizes. And she has kept off those thirty-one pounds for eight years!

Commit Yourself to Change

Did you identify yourself in chapter 2 as needing to lose weight? Did you identify yourself in this chapter as needing a healthier diet?

If so, commit yourself right now to making the changes you need to make. Food is not an enemy, and you're not going to give it up. You're not going to do anything drastic like eating nothing but plain rice, or strawberries and water, or following any of the other fad diets that come and go. These fad diets keep springing up like weeds, and some disappear just as fast.

A fad is any new trend or fashion that suddenly pops up, gets a lot of attention from a zealous band of followers, and then quickly dies out (usually) as its promises clearly remain unfulfilled. Applied to dieting, a fad is any weird or bizarre pattern of eating that usually involves a restricted pattern of allowable foods (sometimes only one) and makes incredible promises about how you will lose weight fast and you will feel better. Such a diet is never based on solid, balanced, scientific evidence and can never deliver what it promises. Usually, it costs a lot of money and makes you feel hungry and uncomfortable, sometimes even sick. Some really extreme fad diets have been so unbalanced that they actually killed people. One of the worst things about most fad diets is that they don't work and may lead to little or no weight loss. And even when loss occurs, it usually is followed by a new weight gain, sometimes going even beyond the original weight to a new, higher weight.

Fad diets do not provide the answer. Don't change your eating habits toward less balance or less variety.

To the contrary, almost everyone needs to develop more balance in his or her diet (we will discuss how in chapter 5). You may need to redirect your appetites. You're not going to try and dam the river of appetite—that's the fad diet way, and it doesn't work for long. If you try to dam up hunger too long, it overflows into a flood of binges. Instead, you're going to rechannel your river of hunger into healthier directions. And soon you will discover that its flow brings you to an unexpected land of zesty, delicious foods you never realized was there before.

Pray to God and ask His wisdom to show you what to change. Ask for His strength to enable you to make that change and stick to it. Remember God's promise: "No temptation [including food] has overtaken you that is not common to man. God is faithful, and he will not let you be tempted beyond your strength, but with the temptation [as to overeat the wrong things] will also provide the way of escape, that you may be able to endure it" (1 Corinthians 10:13).

The fad diet offers you no way out. To avoid temptation, you deprive yourself and suffer. But the GIO-KIO plan *does* offer a way out. When you're tempted to eat the wrong thing, you *don't* simply deny yourself. Instead, you replace the unhealthy item with a healthier one. You *don't* suffer and go hungry!

Some diet books dictate long lists of silly rules you need to follow. Some fad diets want you to eat only one food or one type of food for a certain number of days. Just reading about those diets gives me a sinking feeling in my stomach! I can't imagine trying to live on those diets too long.

But take heart. God made human beings. And He made food. The two go together when coordinated in the right way.

Fad diets are like trying to run your entire home on only one kind of energy. It's silly to think of trying to turn on your electric light bulbs and toaster with a water hose. God's plan matches the different bodily needs with the different food elements that can satisfy those needs. That's like using many different kinds of energy—electrical, gas, thermal—to run the various systems for which they were designed.

And God's plan goes beyond that to give you the power you need to make lasting changes. A fad diet might tell you what to do, but it never tells you *how* to get the power to do it. That's another reason those diets don't work in the long run.

Remember Paul's claim to spiritual power: "I can do all

things in him [Christ] who strengthens me" (Philippians 4:13). That includes gaining control over eating habits.

Make Paul's claim your own. Repeat it every day while you're on the GIO-KIO diet. Repeat it every time you're facing temptation to pour the whipping cream over your strawberries or lather up your roast with extra gravy or coat your toast with so much butter that it drips onto your blouse.

You can control food . . . don't let it control you.

GOD MADE *YOU*

GOD MADE FOOD

LOOK FOR THE *RIGHT* MATCH BETWEEN THE TWO

4

The Purpose of Food

What do you think about food? Circle True or False for each one of the following questions:

T F 1. Sometimes I wish they wouldn't advertise nice-looking food in magazines and on TV.

T F 2. I resent it when people talk about food.

T F 3. If I could just keep food out of the house, I wouldn't want to eat it all the time.

T F 4. Sometimes I get so hungry I can't stand it anymore.

T F 5. I'm determined to lose weight even if it kills me.

T F 6. People who eat a lot make me sick.

T F 7. I've got to stop eating desserts and treats.

T F 8. No matter how skinny everyone else says I am, I know I'm still too fat.

T F 9. If I eat too much, I go make myself vomit so it won't turn to fat.

T F 10. I like to eat in secret so no one else knows how much I'm chowing down.

There's no score or grade on this questionnaire; it's not really a test. But if you circled even one True response, I ask you to read this chapter carefully. Stop to think about what the Bible says concerning food. Try to figure out how and why you developed the attitudes you have. Try to decide if you think they are healthy, or if perhaps you'd like to change your attitudes.

God wants us to have healthy ideas about food, to see its natural role in our lives as He planned it. He wants us to see food as an important gift, but not as the most important one. As the old saying goes, we should "eat to live, not live to eat." In other words, we should eat no more or less than we need to stay healthy and active.

But don't all of us develop some distorted ideas about food? Often we get the wrong idea from the people or the culture around us. We get to thinking either that food is not important and not a good gift from God, or we feel that food and the enjoyment of it matter more than almost anything else in life. Any time we underrate or overvalue food compared to what God thinks about it, we have a distorted idea about food.

Such distorted ideas can lead to food disorders, serious, health-threatening patterns of eating or food avoidance. There is anorexia nervosa, in which the person becomes starved into an emaciated condition. At the other extreme is bulimia, in which the person gorges wildly on food, far beyond normal appetite, and then throws up or otherwise purges himself of the excess food.

Anorexia Nervosa

Sue Ellen is a patient of a clinical nutritionist friend of mine who practices in Boston. When Sue Ellen first began her diet, everything seemed fine. She and her family were delighted with her initial twelve-pound weight loss. She felt younger than her thirty years and basked in the glow of all the favorable comments. But then she decided to quicken the pace. She further cut down her food intake during the week. Some days she would get by on a can of soup and an apple. Then she eliminated food entirely on most weekends. Within a few days, she grew cranky and irritable with her family. She seemed continuously preoccupied and tense at her job as a management intern at a local government bureau. She fell prey to every virus that swept through her office. She often felt weak and tired. When she dipped below 100 pounds, she looked so gaunt and bony that everyone worried about her. Yet she still insisted she was "too fat" and had to keep on her diet "at least a few weeks more."

We usually think of anorexia nervosa as happening to teenage girls. In truth, it does occur mostly among them. But it can also happen to women of other ages and even to men and teenage boys.

Anorexia is a condition like Sue Ellen's in which a person shows an abnormal avoidance of food because she feels she is too fat and must keep losing weight. Sometimes it gets so bad that the person looks like a scrawny victim of starvation. She gets so little protein that her muscles waste away, including those of the heart, making her weak. Growth and development slow down, or even stop altogether. Mental powers fade and moods grow dark and depressed. Sometimes anorexics even die. They have essentially starved themselves past the point of recovery.

This kind of serious neglect of food and normal eating is way off the mark. The person might think, "You can never be too thin," a comment once made by the Duchess of Windsor, who was herself quite trim. But you *can* be too thin. All that self-starvation causes is suffering. It does not honor God, improve health, or increase social popularity.

First Timothy 6:17 tells us that God provides us with everything for our *enjoyment*. He didn't create an infinite variety of foods to tempt us so He could deprive us of them. He didn't create our appetites so we could suppress them and suffer. God is not some big meany way up there in the sky trying to make us miserable.

God created food so that we could *enjoy* it. Don't think that God's diet plan is going to keep you frustrated and starving all the time. We should neither underrate food, failing to appreciate the proper role of balanced food in our lives, nor overrate it, indulging in excess and wild overeating. There is a strong parallel between food and sex. Wild, licentious sex outside of marriage is unhealthy and clearly forbidden in Scripture. But saying that sex is evil and to be avoided at all costs is also unhealthy and unnatural.

Bulimia

In some ways bulimia is the opposite of anorexia. With bulimia the person compulsively overeats rather than starves. (The overeating binge is then followed by a purge.)

But bulimia is similar to anorexia in that with both, the person has a distorted attitude and reaction toward food. And sometimes anorexia can lead to bulimia. This can happen if the intense hunger of anorexia leads to eating binges that then cause guilt so that the person tries to "undo" the damage of overeating.

Leslie is a college girl in her late teens. She had been a popular girl in high school. But it seemed that in college there was more competition for good dates. The boys all seemed to go for those slim, willowy girls. And Leslie had a few extra pounds she wanted to get rid of.

She started dieting. But quickly she got too hungry and weak to keep up with her studies. She really binged one Friday night and ate almost a bag of chips and then a pint of ice cream and a candy bar. She knew that many calories would just start putting back on the weight she had fought so desperately to lose.

Leslie went into the bathroom and made herself throw up all that food. It seemed the perfect solution, at first. She repeated this sequence of gorging and purging more often during the next few months. It seemed she could have the best of both worlds this way: She could enjoy all the pleasures of eating, but she didn't have to worry about slabbing on all that extra weight.

But bulimia is *dangerous*, as Leslie began to find out. She started experiencing depression and feelings of worthlessness. She began to suffer from terrible headaches. And she began to feel the grip of her habit tightening around her life like a noose.

For people with serious or long-term cases of bulimia, the consequences can be severe. The excess eating can cause stomach and intestinal problems such as ulcers, hernias, and even ruptures. Repeated forced vomiting throws off the chemical balance of the body, and the stomach acids can harm the teeth.

Furthermore, this condition shows another perverted view of food. Food was created for our enjoyment. If anorexia is a perverted denial of this fact, bulimia is an exaggerated, unwholesome distortion of it. Again, it's like the difference between love and lust. Enjoying food properly is like enjoying the beauty of sex in a happy marriage. But bulimic binges more closely resemble a pagan orgy.

In fact, the old pagans had something that at first glance resembles bulimia. The ancient Greeks had Epicurus, who once said, "The fountain and root of every good is the pleasure of the stomach."[1] Because of this cultural emphasis on eating as the main pleasure in life, the wealthy began to spend enormous sums on vast and incredibly sumptuous banquets. The chosen guests would feast for days on the most expensive fare known.

The Romans borrowed some of these ideas and went one step further. When they had feasted to the point that they could eat no more, they would force themselves to vomit it all up so that they could go back to eating again. The wealthy would go to the *vomitoria* to gorge and purge, gorge and purge. As the Roman senator Seneca said of that period, "Men eat to vomit and vomit to eat."[2] Some people would squander enormous fortunes on such wasteful and unhealthy extravagance. The main difference between this ancient practice and current bulimia is that bulimics now generally "pig out" and vomit in private, hiding in shame what they are doing. The ancient Romans attending the *vomitoria* did so as a social practice, a kind of wild party.

In short, both extremes—compulsively denying yourself or overly satiating yourself—are unhealthy. Furthermore, vomiting (or using other purge techniques like excessive laxatives) wastes food. (It can be expensive to buy all that food, but that is another matter.)

Food Is *Not* the Enemy

God created food for us to enjoy. Do you remember when He led the Israelites out of their bondage in Egypt? He not only sent them into freedom, He sent them into a land they could *enjoy*. Exodus 3:8 calls it "a land flowing with milk and honey."

Milk and honey taste good. They are nutritious and filling. Yet the Israelites, as they wandered in the wilderness, had not yet reached that wonderful land. Instead of looking forward to it in faith, they complained bitterly about what they had left behind. They relished memories of the food they ate in bondage (Numbers 11:4–6).

I see a powerful metaphor here that applies to most people today. Each of us was raised a little differently. Some grew up in families where we had lots of cake, pie, ice cream, doughnuts, cookies, candy, and other desserts and treats. Some grew up eating loads of high-fat and high-cholesterol foods like bacon, eggs, hot dogs, sausage, and juicy steaks.

However we were raised, we generally associate our past eating habits with good times, a sense of belonging, love, and the sweetness of remembered childhood. One reason we reach for that second ice cream sundae with Dutch chocolate ice cream, syrup, and whipped cream is that eating it makes us feel good psychologically as well as physically. The familiar can be pleasant and comforting.

We should realize that certain of our eating habits are keeping us in bondage to creeping overweight. They are clogging our arteries and threatening to give us heart attacks or strokes. We must be led out of the bondage of poor eating habits.

For a while we are in a transition period in terms of eating. We've left the familiar behind, but we aren't sure of what lies ahead. At times we forget the promise of a brighter future and long for the past again.

This is understandable. We all do it. But we must keep the goal in sight: We do not leave the old habits behind just to wander in the desert of hunger for the rest of our lives. If we look forward in faith, we can enter the promised land of good eating habits, habits that are both healthy and satisfy our hunger.

You can do it, I can do it. In faith, we *can* do it. By taking
Daniel's ten-day diet challenge in chapter 16, you can make the
transition from the old to the new in just ten days. Forty years
of wandering in the wilderness are not required to relearn
healthy eating habits!

Food is not the enemy. But bondage to bad eating habits is.
Start breaking free today.

Food Is a Gift of God

God created food for us to enjoy, yes. But many people take
that out of context to mean that we can freely use food as a sort
of drug: whenever you feel blue, eat; whenever you are upset,
eat; when things don't go your way at work or school, make up
for it with food treats.

But that is *not* what is meant by godly enjoyment of food.
That's another form of self-indulgence. We shouldn't revel in
food and eating as entertainment or recreation or as a means of
getting comfort to recompense us for the trials of daily living.

To enjoy food in the proper sense means to be aware that God
has met our needs, to feel nourished and restored to further serve
God. Or, as Ecclesiastes 3:13 puts it, ". . . it is God's gift to man
that every one should eat and drink and take pleasure in all his
toil."

Once you start thinking of food and eating as a gift, you get a
healthier, more balanced view. Food is not an enemy to avoid;
it is not a lust object to revel in. It is a gift, nothing more,
nothing less. We thank God for this gift and ask His guidance
on how best to enjoy it.

When you use food as a gift from God, not as a crutch or an
escape, food compulsions have no more power over you. You
realize that food is a means to the end of renewing your strength,
not the pleasurable end itself to be pursued at all costs.

Why Fad Diets Are Doomed

A fad diet is one that restricts you to a limited range of foods.
It makes you either avoid foods that are good for you or eat so

much of a given item or two that it becomes too much. A fad diet promises you the world, but doesn't deliver. You'll see it raved about in the media one month, but then hear little or nothing about it again because the diet chasers have already rushed on to the next diet fashion or trend. Such people change their fashions in diet more often than their clothes.

Fad diets go against the grain. They often teach the opposite about food from what the Bible says. Some of them teach that food is an enemy and that we must try to exterminate our appetites. With such teaching it is no wonder that such eating disorders as anorexia and bulimia have reached epidemic proportions.

If you try to live by one of these diets, you are perpetually at war with yourself. The fad diet concept tells you one thing but your body screams another. You experience increasing hunger, frustration, and unhappiness. You cannot deny the natural bodily hunger mechanisms that God created for long. Soon enough, you utterly reject the fad diet.

Worse, you have felt deprived for so long that you usually tend to overcompensate. You eat too much, especially the wrong things. So your approach to food is like a pendulum swinging from one extreme to the other. And your body weight goes up and down like a yo-yo as you jump from one fad diet to another.

Melba is a twenty-nine-year-old married woman. At her peak she weighed 128 pounds, which is too much for someone only five feet tall with a petite body frame. At first she was resistant to making long-term dietary changes because she had suffered through too many fad diets. Says Melba, "I dislike painful dieting—I won't sacrifice what I really want." She had an especially difficult time cutting down on junk food. But when she started consistently changing over to more low-fat foods, she lost twenty-three pounds, ending up with a weight of 105 that she has kept for two years now.

Rather than waste time and money on fad diets and endure cycles of intense hunger followed by regaining all the lost weight plus more, commit yourself to a godly understanding of the body and of food. Then, instead of suffering the worst of

both worlds—hunger and fat—you can enjoy the *best* of both
worlds by eating your fill *and* maintaining a safe, healthy
weight. There is *no* painful dieting on the GIO-KIO plan!

Does this seem impossible? It's not if you are willing to
change your eating habits. You need to put them more in line
with food as God designed. If you fill up on fresh, lean, whole
foods, as God made them, you won't grow obese. But if you
keep filling up on processed foods with concentrated fats, oils,
sweets, and salt, you will put on more fat than you need.

This approach of tuning your habits into eating food as God
designed works. Fifteen years ago, before ever starting a diet, I
reached my peak weight. Once I got on the right track, the fat
just melted away. My weight has fluctuated some since then,
but for fifteen years I have kept it well below the peak I had as
a young man. You can do it, too. The alternative is to keep
seeing your peak weight rise higher year after year.

One of my correspondents told me about her friend Herb.
This poor young man jumps from one fad diet to another. As
my correspondent said, he "is constantly dieting but gains
more weight each year."

Another of my correspondents told me about her aunt who
"starts a new diet every Monday which lasts . . . until Tuesday."

Rather than flying from diet to diet like a bee zipping through
a field of flowers, the smart person will find a *good* diet and
stick to it. You need a diet that recognizes the reality of bodily
needs and the true purpose of foods. You need a diet and health
plan you can stick to *comfortably*, with enjoyment, for the rest
of your life.

FOOD IS NOT THE ENEMY; OVEREATING IS

Section II

Learning How to Eat Right

5

What Is a Good Diet?

It's time now for a complete explanation of the GIO-KIO (Getting It Off, Keeping It Off) plan. This chapter provides the foundation for a good diet that you can live with happily for the rest of your life. And it's much simpler than you might think. After you've read this chapter, you'll realize that the plan boils down to selecting the right foods. And this plan gives you the handful of rules you'll need to do just that. In chapter 16 we'll present Daniel's ten-day diet challenge, with complete menus and recipes for all meals and snacks for the first ten days to get you started right. After that, if you refer back to the basic principles outlined here, you'll be able to make sensible and healthy—not to mention tasty and filling—food selections for the rest of your life.

The key to the diet can be summed up as follows:

- Eat only when you're hungry and *stop eating* when you're not hungry.
- Eat a *variety* of foods.
- Eat mostly whole, *natural* foods, as God designed them.
- Whenever possible, go for a *low-fat* rather than high-fat food.

Eat a Variety of Foods

Many dieters think that the key to losing weight is to reduce the variety of the foods they eat. They might, for example, give up all meat and desserts, eating only fish and rice. Or they might give up all animal foods and eat only fruits and vegetables. I even saw a diet in which you are supposed to eat nothing, for a whole week, except peaches. *Nothing* but peaches. These fad diets don't help much because they teach the opposite of the truth. The vast majority of people need more variety, not less, in their diets. By following the fad diet, you might with effort and suffering lose some weight, but those pounds will surely come back.

Linda is thirty-five years old, single, and a respiratory therapist and Sunday-school teacher. Once she went on a diet plan that called for eating nothing but special food liquids and powders produced by the diet company. She lost three pounds in just two days (from 135 pounds to 132). But she felt "irritable and negative toward life." By the end of the second day she was suffering from tremors and extreme headaches. This terrified her, and she immediately ended the diet. The result? She had lost three pounds, but quickly gained back seven! She had paid good money and risked her health, all for a *net gain of four pounds!*

Then there is Bill, who went on a crash diet for three weeks. He ended up with a net gain of eighteen pounds!

A doctor friend of mine told me about a fifty-five-year-old man who went on a fad diet and ended up as her patient. This particular diet involves total abstinence from protein. After reading chapter 8, I hope you will realize how dangerous something like that can be. As my friend says, the man began to look like a "skeleton" and had to be admitted to the hospital for emergency treatment!

The worst case I know is a woman who wore a size eight when she first became an adult. At that time she weighed about 110 pounds. But then she got scared when she noticed the weight starting to slip on. Panicked, she ran to a diet company. She got into one of those weight-loss programs where you have to purchase most of your food in the form of special products from the company. Over the years she has gained more weight than she lost, and now weighs about 300 pounds! All that time, money, and suffering, and now she has to wear a size twenty!

I'm not saying that all diet products are bad or harmful. Some of them are quite balanced nutritionally. The medical supplements that are produced to feed hospital patients who can't eat normally are wonderful, they help save lives. But for the normal person, *no artificial product can be healthier than a balance of fresh foods, as God designed.*

Let me say that again, because it is important. No food produced artificially can be superior overall to the natural foods that God created. Because an artificial product might have more concentrated vitamins or minerals, balance will be sacrificed, and something else will be left out.

One of the canned liquid protein diets a few years ago, for example, killed dozens of people.[1] It was low calorie and helped them lose weight but it had poor quality protein, and key amino acids were left out. People who forsook real food and stuck only with this product got sick. And some died!

Dr. Philip Felig of the Yale University School of Medicine warns that "all very low-calorie diets are inherently dangerous" even if they do have balanced protein.[2] If you want to experiment with various food supplements and replacements, *which I do not think is a good idea,* I make these recommendations:

1. Don't rely only on the artificial food, no matter what the manufacturer and salesperson say. Keep eating at least some real foods at the same time.
2. At the first sign of adverse physical reaction, cut back on or eliminate the product completely and get back to real food.
3. If you have any doubt whether the resulting physical reaction may be serious, see your physician at once.

With the GIO-KIO diet and health plan you don't need those expensive food replacements. You will eat a balanced, healthy

diet from the wonderful variety of natural foods that God
created as a gift for us.

God's foods are superior for the following reasons:

1. They taste better. No artificial flavors and scents come
   close to the God-designed originals. The artificial ones
   at best remind you of the originals, but can't replace
   them.
2. They are more complete. God's foods are loaded with
   vitamins and minerals and other nutrients that science
   is just now beginning to appreciate.
3. They are more balanced. God's foods have the right
   balance of the different nutrients that better suits our
   bodily needs.

I have no objection to one-a-day-type vitamin and mineral
supplements in pill form, however. Until you learn to get a
truly balanced diet from whole foods, you might want the little
extra insurance those pills provide. Just don't rely on pills,
powder, or cans to the exclusion of real food.

How Does Your Diet Rate for Variety?

Answer each of the following questions by circling the letter
of your response, according to the following scale:

A = rarely or never
B = once or twice a week
C = three or four times a week
D = daily or almost daily

How often do you eat:

1. At least six servings of grain foods, such
   as a slice of bread, a half cup of cereal,
   rice, or pasta, per day?   A B C D
2. Foods made from whole grains?   A B C D
3. Three different vegetables per day?   A B C D
4. Cooked dried beans or peas?   A B C D

5. Spinach, broccoli, or other dark green and leafy vegetables?   A B C D
6. Two or more kinds of fruit or fruit juice per day?   A B C D
7. Two servings of milk products, including cheese or yogurt, per day?   A B C D
8. Two servings of high-protein foods, like meat, eggs, or dried beans, per day?   A B C D

This questionnaire and the following guidelines section were adapted in part from *Dietary Guidelines for Americans*, U. S. Department of Agriculture: Home and Garden Bulletin Number 232-1 (April, 1986).

You might expect that the ideal answer for each of these questions is the first or second column. That's not true in this case. Generally we want more variety, not less. So the ideal answers for these questions all come from the third and fourth columns. Keep in mind the following guidelines:

1. You should eat six servings of bread, cereal, and other grain foods *almost daily*. I know, a lot of fad diets tell you to avoid carbohydrates like bread. Wrong! While most nutritionists recommend that you should get less than 30 percent of your calories from fat and only 12 to 15 percent from protein, they recommend that you should get 55 percent *or more* of your calories from carbohydrates, or grains, fruits, and vegetables.
2. You should eat whole-grain breads and cereals *almost daily*. These provide more fiber than products made from highly refined flour. They also provide more of certain vitamins and minerals than do highly refined grain products, even those fortified with extra nutrients.
3. You should eat three or more different vegetables *almost daily*. Fresh vegetables contain all sorts of vitamins and minerals, as well as fiber and digestible carbohydrates. It is possible that they contain nutrients

not yet recognized as such by medical science. (Remember, a lot of the nutrients you read about and that are included in vitamin pills now were not recognized as nutrients ten or twenty years ago. There could well be more discoveries in the future. Until this knowledge is complete, artificial supplements will always be inferior to whole, natural foods.)

4. You should eat beans or peas *three to four times a week*. These have good protein without all the animal fat and cholesterol we associate with meat.

5. You should eat spinach or other dark green leafy vegetables *three to four times a week*. These vegetables contain vitamins A and C, riboflavin, and folic acid. They contain the minerals calcium, iron, magnesium, and potassium. A lot of diets are low in some of these nutrients, probably because many people skip these foods almost completely.

6. You should consume two kinds of fruit *almost daily*. I would recommend three or even more kinds of fruit every day. I think most people have drastically reduced their intake of these natural fruits in favor of baked goods and other manufactured sweets. Both taste sweet, but fruit has far more fiber and far less fat than produced candies, ice creams, and bakery items. For instance, one whole orange has only sixty calories and less than one gram of fat. A single Danish pastry with fruit, on the other hand, has 235 calories and *thirteen grams of fat*. Hey, I like Danish, too. By all means, eat some. But don't eat these kinds of sweets only, to the exclusion of fruit. Let's keep our diets in balance.

7. You should have two servings of dairy products *almost daily*. (Teenagers and pregnant or breast-feeding women should eat three servings per day.) For those who suffer from lactose intolerance, or the inability to digest milk sugar (drinking too much milk gives them gas and discomfort), minimize your intake of fluid milk, but go instead for yogurt, cheese, cottage cheese, sour cream, and other milk products. These products almost

never bother people who suffer from lactose intolerance. Because whole milk and milk products have lots of fat, try to go for skim milk or low-fat milk products whenever possible.

8. You should have two servings of high-protein foods *almost daily*. Most Americans get too much rather than too little protein. Instead of four or five servings of such foods a day, try to keep it down to two. Select lean, low-fat versions of protein foods. Stop being overreliant on meat, and try the complementary-protein vegetable combinations to be discussed in chapter 8, such as macaroni and cheese, beans and rice, and so on.

Go back and compare your scores. How does your diet rate for balance and variety? Start changing your eating habits to move your scores closer to the optimum ones. For any item in which your answer was two or more columns away, take immediate action *now* to improve your diet. For instance, on question 6, if you put the first or second columns, and the best answer is column 4, start thinking today about how you can get more fresh fruit into your diet.

What the Bible Says

God didn't create just two or three kinds of food for us. He created a wonderfully rich variety. For centuries, however, the Hebrews developed lists of foods they considered "clean" and thus okay and other foods they considered "unclean," and thus forbidden. This distinction was based in part on animals like the pig, which Leviticus 11 warned them to avoid. But in Mark 7:19 we are told that Jesus declared all foods clean.

Do you remember in Acts 10:9–16 when Peter became hungry and fell into a trance? He had a vision of a large sheet coming down to earth from heaven that contained all sorts of animals, reptiles, and birds. God told Peter to eat one of them and he balked. He said *no way!* He thought it was unclean. But then the voice from heaven told him, "What God has cleansed, you must not call common" (Acts 10:15).

This passage has some important spiritual meanings, but I also see a dietary lesson here. Doesn't it remind you a bit of the mother who prepares a nice dinner and spreads it on the table, only to be told by her kids, "Yuck! I'm not going to eat *that!*" Do we also sometimes treat God that way? Do we focus on two or three of our favorite kinds of food and ignore the rest of the healthful feast that God offers? Let's look at the rich variety that God has provided.

In Genesis 1:29 we read, "And God said, 'Behold, I have given you every plant yielding seed which is upon the face of all the earth, and every tree with seed in its fruit; you shall have them for food.' " God's first gift of food was all sorts of fruits and vegetables.

Then in Genesis 9:3, after the flood, God says to Noah and his sons, "Every moving thing that lives shall be food for you; and as I gave you the green plants, I give you everything." God's second gift of food was all varieties of animal life, both land animals and seafood.

In various places the Bible mentions such foods as bread, butter, cheese, dried and fresh fruit, fish, honey, locusts, meat, milk, oil, quail, and vegetables. All these except locusts sound fairly familiar to us today. Our society does not look favorably on insects; the thought of them as food doesn't make our mouths water. Yet people in other cultures prize certain insects for food, including certain kinds of worms.[3] I have heard of people even in America who apparently like to eat worms (personally, I draw the line at that point). Nevertheless we should consider 1 Timothy 4:4: "For everything created by God is good, and nothing is to be rejected if it is received with thanksgiving."

Guidelines for Achieving Dietary Balance

In a later chapter I will give you enough menus to last for the period of Daniel's ten-day diet challenge so you can get a feel for the marvelous benefits of a strict diet. If you find that sample diet too stringent for you beyond ten days, you may want to widen your food choices more afterward, as Daniel himself did. Once you gain a basic understanding of the dietary balance principle, which we'll discuss more here, you will be able to wisely select low-fat foods for a proper balance to your diet.

By following these simple guidelines you will be able to expand your food choices to include all the kinds of food you already know and love and, hopefully, many new ones as well. For instance, if the plan calls for a serving of meat, you can choose roast beef one day, a pork chop another day, and a lamb chop or roast ham on another day. You can select any food you like as long as you substitute one from the same category. In other words, substitute any meat for a meat selection, any fruit for a fruit selection, and so on. It's not the exact foods that count so much as fulfilling the need for variety among the categories of food.

Here are the guidelines to follow in selecting the right numbers of servings of each kind of food. Also included are the relative amounts of each kind you should eat. The actual item you choose in each category doesn't matter that much as long as you cover all the categories each day with the right numbers of servings. The Weekly Food Planner and Diary will help you keep track of what you eat.

1. *High-protein foods.* Each day, try to get two or three servings of these foods: meat, poultry, fish, eggs, beans, peas, and nuts. *Do not* eat a lot more than that on a regular basis. Try to keep these items as lean and fat-free as possible: for example, trim away excess fat. Try to avoid more than one animal protein food in a given meal, except on special occasions. For instance, *don't* eat eggs and bacon and sausage in the same meal, at least not on a routine basis. In terms of serving sizes, your total daily intake of meat, fish, or poultry should be no more than about five ounces for a woman or seven ounces for a man. Except for special occasions, forget about those sixteen- or twenty-one-ounce steaks for a single meal. (You could always eat half and take the rest home for another day.) Avoid more than two or three eggs a week, because egg yolks are one of the highest known sources of cholesterol and other fats.

Weekly Food Planner and Diary

	High-Protein Foods	Dairy Products	Grain Products		Vege-tables	Fruit
Sunday	☐___ ☐___ ☐___	☐___ ☐___	☐___ ☐___ ☐___ ☐___ ☐___	☐___ ☐___ ☐___ ☐___ ☐___	☐___ ☐___ ☐___	☐___ ☐___ ☐___
Monday	☐___ ☐___ ☐___	☐___ ☐___	☐___ ☐___ ☐___ ☐___ ☐___	☐___ ☐___ ☐___ ☐___ ☐___	☐___ ☐___ ☐___	☐___ ☐___ ☐___
Tuesday	☐___ ☐___ ☐___	☐___ ☐___	☐___ ☐___ ☐___ ☐___ ☐___	☐___ ☐___ ☐___ ☐___ ☐___	☐___ ☐___ ☐___	☐___ ☐___ ☐___
Wednesday	☐___ ☐___ ☐___	☐___ ☐___	☐___ ☐___ ☐___ ☐___ ☐___	☐___ ☐___ ☐___ ☐___ ☐___	☐___ ☐___ ☐___	☐___ ☐___ ☐___
Thursday	☐___ ☐___ ☐___	☐___ ☐___	☐___ ☐___ ☐___ ☐___ ☐___	☐___ ☐___ ☐___ ☐___ ☐___	☐___ ☐___ ☐___	☐___ ☐___ ☐___
Friday	☐___ ☐___ ☐___	☐___ ☐___	☐___ ☐___ ☐___ ☐___ ☐___	☐___ ☐___ ☐___ ☐___ ☐___	☐___ ☐___ ☐___	☐___ ☐___ ☐___
Saturday	☐___ ☐___ ☐___	☐___ ☐___	☐___ ☐___ ☐___ ☐___ ☐___	☐___ ☐___ ☐___ ☐___ ☐___	☐___ ☐___ ☐___	☐___ ☐___ ☐___

2. *Dairy products.* Have at least two servings a day of milk, cheese, or yogurt. (Women who are pregnant or breast-feeding should eat more.) Dairy products provide both valuable protein and one of our richest sources of calcium, the mineral important for bones and teeth. In terms of serving sizes, count one cup of milk, one cup of yogurt, and about two ounces of cheese as one serving.

3. *Grain products.* Have six to ten servings a day of bread, cereal, pasta, rice, and other grain products. Several or even most of these servings should be whole grain, that is, dark bread rather than white bread, dark cereals rather than refined, airy ones. Count as one serving each slice of bread, each half of a bun or muffin, two large crackers, one-half cup of cooked cereal, rice, or pasta, and one ounce of packaged breakfast cereal.

4. *Vegetables.* Have three to five servings each day. Try to encompass the different kinds of vegetables every day. Instead of five leafy, green vegetables, try leafy green vegetables *and* yellow ones, starchy ones like potatoes, and legumes like beans and peas. (Legumes also count as a protein item, so you can kill two birds with one stone.) Whenever possible, eat raw vegetables: for example, carrot sticks, celery, cauliflower, mixed salads with lettuce, tomato, spinach, cucumber, radishes, mushrooms, onions, green peppers, and so on. Certain vegetables like corn and potatoes, however, taste better cooked to most people. For variety take several salad ingredients and stir-fry them in a tiny bit of oil for a Chinese-style dish. Reduce your intake of canned vegetables, because some nutrients are lost due to processing and time in storage. Count as one serving one cup of leafy raw vegetables like lettuce, but only one-half cup of chopped or cooked vegetables.

5. *Fruit.* Try to have two to four servings every day, preferably of fresh items whenever possible. And again, go for variety each day. Don't just have four apples but try for one apple, banana, orange, and pear. Count each

whole fruit as one serving, but count grapefruit as two. Count as one serving a melon wedge, one-half cup cooked fruit, one-half cup berries, one-quarter cup dried fruit, three-quarters cup juice. Get no more than half your daily servings of fruit as juice. It contains many of the important vitamins, but it lacks fiber (roughage) and the mouth-watering satisfaction you get by chewing on a sweet, tasty fruit.

6. *Try to avoid extra salt, fat* (e.g., butter, salad dressing), *sugar, alcoholic beverages, and highly refined sweets and baked goods.* Some is okay, but fill up first with the healthy stuff just mentioned, and top off with just a bit of dessert. Don't skip solid items to leave a lot of room for a pile of treats.

7. *Go for variety in cooking styles.* Try fresh and cooked, steamed, grilled, baked, broiled, and stir-fried. However, try to avoid techniques that involve a lot of fat, especially deep-fat frying. Cooking foods in fat makes them absorb more fat. And fat not only is the most concentrated source of calories in the food supply, but an excess of it poses a number of health risks (more on this in chapter 6).

8. *Herbs and spices.* Jazz up your dishes and add more diversity to your menu by flavoring food items and combinations in different ways. We'll spend more time on this topic later, in chapter 9.

Seeking out variety in your menu helps you to lose weight and at the same time keeps you healthy, strong, and vigorous. Melinda, who is twenty-eight and single, weighed in at 118 pounds before starting the program. Although this does not represent much overweight, in Melinda's own words, her goal was "to be five to eight pounds lighter." Rather than diminish the variety of the foods she ate, she wisely cut down serving sizes. She especially was concerned about reducing her intake of chocolate and ice cream. As a result, in just two weeks she lost five pounds, declining to 113. Even more exciting than the missing pounds, she reports that with a solid variety in her diet she feels great, better than ever. She has experienced an increased energy level, feels better about herself, and is peppy and more self-confident.

That's the way you will feel, too, when you get started with this plan and introduce yourself to the wide variety of foods that God has so richly bestowed on us. Eating right not only helps you lose fat and get down to your natural, ideal body weight, it also makes you more healthy and provides the energy and the vigor you need to cope with the demands of a busy life.

Where fad diets leave you weak, cranky, and with strong hunger cravings, God's diet plan leaves you full, satisfied, happy, and stronger than ever before. You will feel the difference in your own body, you will see the difference in the mirror, and you will enjoy the difference in your mind. You will have more power to get through your daily life.

For Healthy Hearts: Balance Your Family's Diet!

Eat More of These	Moderate Amounts of These	Less of These
	MILK, CHEESE, BUTTER, OIL	
Nonfat fortified milk; skim milk; low-fat yogurt; buttermilk (made with skim milk); low-fat cottage cheese; cheeses containing less than 5% butterfat; margarine (soft tub or stick made with corn, cottonseed, soy, safflower or sunflower oils *only*); corn oil; sunflower oil; safflower oil; peanut oil; soy oil	1% or 2% fat-fortified milk; frozen yogurt; low-fat, hard cheese; ice milk; soft margarine; mayonnaise; skimmed, evaporated milk (good for cooking in place of cream or whole milk)	Whole and chocolate milk; canned, evaporated whole milk; buttermilk; whole cream; hard and cream cheeses; sour cream; high-fat ice cream; butter; shortening; lard; bacon fat; eggs

MEAT, FISH, POULTRY

Fresh or fresh-frozen fish; tuna; crab; scallops; chicken, turkey, cornish hen (without the skin); lean veal	(Trim off fat) Flank steak; beef filet; leg of lamb; sirloin; pork (whole rump center shank); ham (center slices); rib eye; ground beef; pork loin; boiled ham; chicken frankfurter	(Trim off fat) Corned beef (brisket); hamburger (commercial); steaks (club and rib); rib roast; breast of lamb; spareribs; ground pork; deviled ham; breast of veal; regular frankfurter; cold cuts; fried chicken (with skin or prepared with saturated oil); duck and goose; sausage and bacon; liver, heart, and other organ meats; sardines

VEGETABLES

(Fresh is best, raw or steamed) Asparagus; bean sprouts; beets; broccoli; brussels sprouts; cauliflower; cabbage; carrots; eggplant; green beans; string beans; squash (summer); zucchini; cucumbers; watercress; lettuce; corn; peas	Canned vegetables (some are high in salt, check label); frozen vegetables (without added salt); canned vegetable soups (read label for salt content); stir-fried vegetables prepared in small amount of polyunsaturated fat	Vegetables fried in butter or other saturated fats; frozen vegetables (processed with salt, such as mixed vegetables); vegetables made with cream and butter sauces

FRUITS, FRUIT JUICES

Apples/apple juice; apricots (fresh or dried); bananas; berries; cherries; dates; figs; grapes; oranges; peaches; plums; grapefruit; prunes; raisins; fresh fruit juices without added sugar	Fruits canned in juices; fruits canned in water; fruit ice;	Fruits canned in heavy syrup; fruit drinks; glazed fruit (all fruits to which sodium, coloring or sodium benzoate has been added)

STARCHES, CEREALS, GRAINS

Whole wheat, rye, pumpernickel, raisin breads; cornmeal; whole wheat pasta; brown rice; potatoes (sweet or white); yams; pumpkin; beans and lentils; grits; wheat germ; oatmeal; puffed rice

White bread; refined pasta; white rice; refined, unsweetened cereal; low-salt whole wheat crackers made with soybean oil

Instant potatoes; other prepared potato products (these are high in salt); french fries; commercially prepared foods such as macaroni and cheese, lasagna, pizza, cheese blintzes (homemade foods are better); sweetened cereal; sweet rolls; salted crackers made with palm and/or coconut oil

SNACKS, DESSERTS, NUTS

Fresh fruits and vegetables; dried fruits (raisins); low-fat yogurt; popcorn (unsalted, unbuttered); homemade oatmeal cookies (made with safflower, cottonseed, or corn oil, raisins and raw apples)

Low-fat or part-skim cheeses; ice milk; peanut butter; unsalted peanuts; walnuts; almonds; pecans (fat content is mainly monounsaturated)

Commercial cakes; cookies; pies; candy; ice cream; soda; potato and corn chips; salted peanuts; pretzels

DRESSINGS, SAUCES, CONDIMENTS

Natural herbs and spices; fresh onion; garlic powder; pepper; lemon juice; tomato; lettuce; onion; cucumber

Unsalted, low-fat salad dressing; homemade dressing made with polyunsaturated oils (safflower, corn, or cottonseed)

All are high in salt: steak sauces; soy sauce; salt; garlic, celery and onion salts; meat tenderizers; celery seed; horseradish; commercial salad dressings; salted meat gravy; chili sauce; butter sauces

This chart is taken from *Pediatric Nutrition Highlights* (Philadelphia: Wyeth Laboratories, 1984), p. 4.

How to Satisfy Your Hunger Right Now

In a later chapter I'm going to give you a complete ten-day
menu plan so you'll learn exactly how to make the right food
choices. This will be something like what I imagine Daniel put
together for his diet challenge with the Babylonian menu.

But let's say that you don't want to wait ten more chapters to
see what you can eat. You've been reading about food for some
pages now, and all this food talk is making you hungry. The
chocolate chip cookies in the kitchen cabinet are starting to
sing out to you. You want a snack and you want it *now*. Do you
believe that we can fill up your stomach right now without
adding to your fat?

I've already said that you don't have to give up all your
favorite foods, like desserts. But I do want you to start giving up
rich, fatty, and sweet desserts *as snacks*. Don't panic—you can
have some cheesecake or French apple pie tonight for dessert.
But let's get rid of desserts for your between-meal snacks. Here
are the foods I want you to *avoid as snacks*:

Dairy: chocolate milk, condensed milk, eggnog, milk
    shakes, ice cream
Pastries: cakes (except angel or sponge cake), doughnuts,
    pies, cookies, sweet rolls
Cereals: those sweetened with sugar (some packaged
    cereals consist of as much as 50 percent sugar)

Instead of eating desserts as snacks, we're going to try some
of Daniel's food for snacks. Try eating some of these raw. If you
want a little extra flavor, add vinegar, lemon juice, or a sprinkle
of salt, but not a creamy dip.

carrots	lettuce (iceberg or romaine)
cauliflower	mushrooms
celery	parsley
chicory	radishes
Chinese cabbage	spinach
cucumber	tomatoes
endive	watercress
escarole	

Most of these foods are so low in calories that the act of eating
them almost burns up the calories that you consume. The next
time you get the munchies, take your fill of any of these
vegetables or the following list of foods. And don't forget about
unbuttered popcorn, my personal favorite. That's good any
time. Another good idea is to take a big drink of water any time
you feel hungry. Water helps you feel full faster when you do
begin to eat. The following is a list of unlimited free foods.

bouillon	lemon juice (unsweetened)
clear broth (fat-free)	lime juice (unsweetened)
cranberries	pickles (unsweetened)
gelatin, unsweetened	spices
gum, sugar-free	soft drinks (sugar-free)
herbs	

(*Caution:* If you tend toward high blood pressure, avoid too
much salt, soy sauce, and other salty condiments.)

Do you see anything on those two lists that you like? If you're
hungry, put the book down right now and go have a snack.
Enjoy yourself. Eat your fill. Eat slowly and relish every bite.
Thank God for giving you tangy, zesty foods that taste good, feel
good in your mouth, and satisfy that empty feeling in your
stomach.

You can snack on any of these foods any time you want, day
or night. Don't worry if it's just before dinner time or bedtime.
If you're hungry, you're hungry. You won't have peace of mind
about your diet until you get beyond aching physical hunger.

If your stomach is empty, it's too easy to dream about that
vanilla fudge or strawberry shortcake. But when your stomach
is full of healthy foods that give you energy, zip, and that
wide-awake feeling, you won't miss fatty sweets. Anyway, you
can have some of that candy or cake later today, too. Just don't
pig out on it.

This approach of relying on healthy snacks rather than sweet
dessert-type snacks works. Neil is a thirty-three-year-old respiratory therapist who followed my advice about eating lots of
vegetables. He especially enjoyed fresh homemade coleslaw.

And this diet worked well for him. He dropped thirteen pounds in just eight weeks. And he *kept* it off for seven years.

You can do it, too. Remember, ". . . whether you eat or drink, or whatever you do, do all to the glory of God" (1 Corinthians 10:31).

VARIETY
IN YOUR DIET
EQUALS
POWER
IN YOUR BODY

Avoid Excess Fat

Avoiding excess fat is one of the key principles in the GIO-KIO diet plan. Remember, you have to eat fat to put on fat. Once you start reducing your fat intake, the fat of *your own body will begin to disappear.* You will burn it right off!

Daniel avoided the fat, greasy foods of the Babylonians and in ten days he looked a miracle of health compared to the young men who gorged on lard and cholesterol. The day you begin to cut down on your fat intake, that same day you will begin to feel more alive, stronger, and healthier. Within days you'll notice the needle on the bathroom scale going down and people will tell you how much better you look. Soon you'll be buying a new set of clothes, in much smaller sizes.

Karen is forty-seven years old, married, and an active church member. She used to weigh 252 pounds, about 100 pounds more than she should. However, once she started cutting down on fatty foods, she lost 50 pounds in just six months. She kept that off for two years. Now she says, "I am committed to losing another 50 to 60 pounds and *finally*—after more than twenty years—weighing what I should."

I know a man who was dangerously obese until he also cut down on fat intake. *He lost 200 pounds.* And he has kept it off for five years! The experience of gaining control over his life meant so much to him that he is planning to work as a counselor for overweight teens.

Beware of Eating Too Much Fat

It takes fat to make fat because fat is the most concentrated source of calories. In other words, the more fat you eat, the more likely you are to put more body fat onto your frame.

Before studying nutrition in school, I had many misconceptions about where fat was in food. There is, of course, the easily visible fat that you see on slices of ham, beef, and other meats. I always used to trim that off, so I thought I ate little fat indeed.

It *is* a good idea to trim off visible fat. But it's the kind you don't see that is more prevalent and more likely to do you in. For example, you don't see the fat in peanuts, yet an ounce of roasted peanuts has about 165 calories, 76 percent due to fat. Three-quarters of the energy in peanuts is due to fat!

Fats include all sorts of oils and greases as well as solid, visible fat. Any one of the following contains five grams of fat and forty-five calories:

Avocado	⅛	(4″ diameter)
Bacon, crisp	1	slice
Bacon fat	1	teaspoon
Butter or margarine	1	teaspoon
Margarine, dietetic	2	teaspoons
Cream		
Heavy	1	tablespoon
Light	2	tablespoons
Sour	2	tablespoons
Cream cheese	1	tablespoon
Dressing		
French	1	tablespoon
Italian	1	tablespoon
Mayonnaise	1	teaspoon
Roquefort	2	teaspoons

Russian	2	teaspoons
Salad dressing		
(Mayonnaise type)	2	teaspoons
Sandwich spread	1	tablespoon
Thousand Island	2	teaspoons
Gravy	2	tablespoons
Lard	1	teaspoon
Nuts		
Almonds	10	whole
Peanuts, Spanish	20	whole
Peanuts, Virginia	10	whole
Pecans	2	large, whole
Walnuts	6	small
Others	6	small
Oil or cooking fat	1	teaspoon
Olives	5	small
Pork, salt	¾″	cube
Seeds, hulled	1	tablespoon

Source: Your Calorie Diet (Washington, D. C.: Department of the Army, 1977), pp. 33–34.

Do You Eat Too Much Fat?

We'll talk more about dietary fats later. Right now fill out this little questionnaire so you can see if you eat too much fat. Circle the letter corresponding to how often you eat each kind of food, using this scale:

A = rarely or never
B = one or two times a week
C = three to five times a week
D = daily or almost daily

How often do you eat:

1. Fried or breaded foods?   A B C D

   2. Processed meats like sausage or cold cuts,
      fatty meats like bacon, and steaks or roasts
      with lots of visible fat?   A B C D
   3. Dairy products made with whole milk,
      including ice cream and cheese?   A B C D
   4. Rich desserts like pies, cakes, and other
      pastries?   A B C D
   5. Rich sauces and gravies?   A B C D
   6. Regular salad dressings or mayonnaise? A B C D
   7. Products containing rich cream, e.g.,
      whipped cream or sour cream?   A B C D
   8. Butter or margarine?   A B C D

Adapted from *Dietary Guidelines for Americans,* U. S. Department of Agriculture: Home and Garden Bulletin Number 232–3 (April, 1986), p. 1.

All the foods on this list are high in fat. For instance, you start with a piece of fish that has less than 100 calories per portion. If you boil it or bake it plain, it will stay that way. But if you bread it and fry it in oil or another fat, the breading and fish surface can absorb hundreds of calories in fat.

I love the taste of hot dogs as much as any kid frolicking at the beach. But I restrict myself to few per month because 81 percent of the calories in a hot dog are due to fat! In processed lunch meats you don't see the fat as clearly as on a roast or steak. But it's there.

Dairy products based on whole milk or cream have loads of fat. Basically, the cream has the fat. To produce low-fat milk and dairy products, a certain amount of the cream is removed, leaving the water, protein, and other nutrients. Desserts, gravies, salad dressings, butter, margarine, and other foods using a lot of oil, cream, or meat drippings are loaded with fat.

Don't get too worried if you see all or almost all of your favorite foods on the list. This is *not* a forbidden list. No one is going to tell you to avoid every food on it. God created meat, milk, nuts, and other high-fat foods for a reason. He gave them to us for food. In fact, certain fatty acids (components of fat) are *essential to life.* In other words, you must eat some fat or you will die.

It's not a matter of saying yes or no to fatty foods. It's a question of how much and how often.

Look back at your answers on the questionnaire. Anything you marked in the first two columns is fine. Now, you shouldn't have too many items in column three. If you have more than four items in that column, I'd start to think about cutting down.

If you have anything in the fourth column, you definitely should consider cutting it down. But don't worry. You are not going to give it up and go hungry. You won't suffer a sense of deprivation. Later we're going to talk about replacing these give-ups with a lot of really tasty give-in-tos.

You see, it's the balance of your diet that is so important. Nutritionists estimate that the average American gets about 40 to 50 percent of his or her calories as fat. That's way too much. The American Heart Association recommends that you get no more than 30 percent of your calories as fat.[1] For every hot dog at 81 percent you've got to add some good items like peaches (0 percent fat) or French bread (9 percent fat). That will bring down your average to a more reasonable figure.

Why Food Has So Much Fat

The simple reason that we eat too much fat is that it tastes good. It is filling. And knowing this, livestock farmers, food manufacturers, and other food dealers tend to put extra fat into our food supply.

Cattle are now bred and fed to produce a lot more fat than most animals in Bible times did. Commercially prepared sauces and gravies usually have lots of fat (as well as sugar and salt). The simple plain potato has almost no fat; but instead of eating it plain, we eat it as chips, fries, or various other snacks that have hundreds of fat calories added due to cooking that poor little potato in fats and oils.

I like potato chips as much as the next guy. *They do taste good*, and as the ad says, it's hard "to eat just one." But I try to cut down on consumption of these fatty alternatives by filling up on whole, fresh foods instead.

We should all try to resist the temptation to eat the forbidden fruit of excess fat. Leviticus 3:17 says, "It shall be a perpetual statute throughout your generations, in all your dwelling places, that you eat neither fat nor blood." Leviticus 7:23 adds, "... You shall eat no fat, of ox, or sheep, or goat." These verses are talking about visible strips of fat, of course, because it is basically impossible to remove all fat from food (except by laboratory means that alter completely the nature of the food).

The Bible has always warned us against eating too much animal fat. Yet science has not discovered until this century the chemical nature of fat, how it interacts in the body, and how it can help cause or worsen disease.

What *Is* Fat?

Fat is the most concentrated source of energy of any food substance. One ounce of pure fat contains approximately 255 calories. (By contrast, an ounce of plain cooked rice contains about 28 calories.) You could spend several minutes enjoying a whole bowl of rice for the same calories as an ounce of fat. Yet you could slurp down the fat in just a moment. Think about it: For the same amount of calories, you could enjoy eating more of a nonfat food for longer than a high-fat food.

Chemically speaking, a molecule of fat consists of glycerol attached to one or more fatty acids. There are three kinds of fatty acids, which you probably have heard of before.

1. *Saturated fatty acids.* These are most common in animal foods and products, though coconut oil and certain other vegetable fats also contain these. Saturated fatty acids are the most unhealthy fats of all. No wonder the Bible warns us away from animal fat!

2. *Monounsaturated fatty acids.* These are found in certain plant and animal foods, for example, olive oil and peanut oil. These are less dangerous than saturated fatty acids.

3. *Polyunsaturated fatty acids.* These are found mostly in plant fats such as corn oil and soybean oil. If you're

going to eat fat, these are the safer ones to have as far as your heart is concerned.

A convenient rule of thumb is that the more saturated the fat, the more likely it is to be solid at room temperature (e.g., lard). A less saturated fat is more likely to be in the liquid state at room temperature (e.g., a vegetable oil). However, despite differences in saturation, all three fats have the same amount of calories per ounce. Thus eating any of them tends to worsen your weight problem.

The total amount of fat you eat can be hazardous even if you eat a good balance of polyunsaturated to saturated fats. In general, we need to get the proportion of our calories eaten as fat down to 30 percent or less.

Health Hazards of Excess Fat in the Diet

Remember, some fat in the diet is okay and even essential. A certain amount of fat is *required* to produce some hormones, cell membranes, and the special sheaths that cover and protect many nerves. We need fat to help us absorb the so-called fat-soluble vitamins (A, D, E, and K). But let's face it, the average person gets way over the minimum requirement of fat he or she really needs. If you're eating lots of fat every day, you could be in trouble. The fat you eat or the fat it leads to in your body is associated with an entire host of diseases:

- *Increased blood pressure (hypertension)*. The more body mass your circulatory system must supply, the harder the heart must work. This raises blood pressure.
- *Increased chance of strokes*. Hypertension can increase the likelihood that you will get a stroke, which can lead to serious brain damage or even death.
- *Atherosclerosis*. High fat intake can lead to increased clogging of the arteries, which can lead to heart attacks.
- *Kidney disease*.
- *Adult diabetes*. This begins most often (but not always)

in overweight people, especially as they approach middle age.

- *Gallstones.* The gallbladder holds the bile that is required for digestion of fats. Eating too much fat or being fat can strain the system.
- *Cancer, especially colon, rectal, and prostate cancer in men, or uterine, bile-duct, and breast cancer in women.* Not only does excess fat help cause breast cancer, one of the most common cancers for women, but after someone develops it, excess dietary fat makes it worse. Among women who have breast cancer, for every extra 1000 grams of fat eaten per month, the risk of death increases by about 50 percent.[2] This means that eating even an extra 30 grams of fat a day could seriously shorten a breast cancer victim's life. And it is so easy to add up an extra 30 grams of fat. Try two eggs fried in butter (14 grams), three slices of bacon (9 grams), and a glass of whole milk (8 grams), and you've got it all just at breakfast!

I hope this dreadful list of diseases caused and worsened by excess dietary fat convinces you that too much fat in the diet *is bad for you.* The typical person in America and Europe eats too much fat, and alarming rates of the various diseases I've referred to have been noted in these regions.

But don't give up hope. The Bible warned us thousands of years ago against too much fat. I'm going to give you fifteen rules to help you heed that warning. Remember, even if you've been eating excess fat for thirty or fifty or more years, *the day you start cutting down is the day you'll start reducing your risk of getting one of these dreaded diseases.* Cut down today!

Fifteen Rules for Avoiding Excess Fat

1. Choose lean cuts of meat. The cheaper kinds of ground beef have much more fat than the more expensive ones. But lean hamburger is still a good buy because you don't lose so much in cooking.

2. Trim visible fat from meat before and after cooking. Don't use it for human consumption, just throw it out.

3. Avoid excess fat when cooking. You should usually avoid *frying* meat, poultry, or fish, especially deep-fat frying. Frying adds loads of fat calories to the surface of whatever is being cooked that way. Instead, roast, bake, broil, or simmer.

4. For poultry, remove the skin before cooking. Most of the fat is connected to the skin.

5. Any form of cooking meat tends to make it ooze fat in the form of meat juices. As a rule, drain off this fat and don't use it. When you bake or broil meat, place it on a rack so the juices produced during cooking will drain off rather than baste back in. Always avoid deliberate basting with fatty juices or pastes. After cooking drain all the fat you can from the meat and get rid of it. Let bacon or burgers drain on paper towels after cooking, to get rid of all the fat possible. This grease is loaded with saturated fat, the worst kind you can eat. Also don't use the same oil or fat repeatedly for cooking after it begins to change color. Heating fats can produce undesirable chemical changes. If you reuse and reheat them, you can produce unacceptable levels of these changes.

6. If you need to save the meat juice or broth for a recipe instead of throwing it out, chill it in the refrigerator first. This solidifies the fat into white blotches which you can remove by hand. The rest of the meat juice turns into a kind of gelatin, which contains protein rather than fat (this is low-quality protein, however).

7. Try to avoid frying vegetables in butter or other fats. Instead, steam, boil, or bake vegetables. If you want to fry, stir fry them in a *small* amount of vegetable oil.

8. Instead of butter or fatty sauces, season cooked vegetables with herbs and spices. These are fat-free and practically calorie-free. (We'll cover specific types of herbs and spices in chapter 9.)

9. Instead of pouring rich, fatty salad dressings on fresh

salads, use lemon juice, small amounts of oil and vinegar, or small portions of low-calorie dressings. Once you stop smothering salads in thick dressing, you'll be amazed at how zesty greens and other salad materials taste naturally. (See the recipe section in chapter 16 for a homemade salad dressing that is practically fat-free and low in calories.)

10. Try to avoid baking with saturated fats such as butter or solid shortening. Margarine and liquid oils contain less saturated fats.

11. Try whole-grain flours to improve the taste of baked goods so that you can use less fat in baking.

12. Use low-fat or skim milk rather than whole milk or cream whenever possible. For coffee and tea use a cream substitute. But avoid those which use coconut oil, for that fat is even more saturated than normal milk cream.

13. In recipes that include sour cream, mayonnaise, or thickened cream, try to substitute low-fat yogurt, or low-fat cottage cheese whipped in your blender, to give it the right consistency.

14. Try to eat no more than three eggs a week, including those used in baked goods or other dishes.

15. If you must use more than three eggs a week, try to stick with the whites, for they have more protein than fat, whereas the yolk has most of the fat.

These rules were adapted in part from *Dietary Guidelines for Americans*, U. S. Department of Agriculture: Home and Garden Bulletin Number 232–3 (April, 1986), p. 8.

Substitutions for High-Fat Foods

This plan does not require you simply to give up yummy foods. In the first place, you can eat some of anything you like, but cut down the quantity if it's a high-fat item. And second, you can substitute a low-fat item for any high-fat one that you're giving up.

As you look at these calorie figures, realize that for each 3500 calories extra that you eat, you put one pound of body fat onto your waist and thighs.

The opposite is also true. For every 3500 calories less that you eat than your body needs, you can *lose* a pound. In other words, if you could cut down 500 calories a day, you could lose a pound of fat a week. (Just estimate this roughly; we *do not* count calories on the GIO-KIO plan.)

Here are some examples of where you can cut down:

Instead Of	Try This	And Save This Many Calories
Whole milk	skim milk	85 per 8-ounce glass
Cream and sugar	artificials	110 per cup of coffee
Chocolate malt	lemonade	400 per 8-ounce glass
Butter	apple butter	80 per slice of toast
Cheesecake	watermelon	140 per slice
Ice cream	yogurt	180 per 8-ounce serving
Apple pie	tangerine	305 per serving
Tuna fish	crabmeat	85 per 3-ounce serving
Fish sticks	plain fish	95 per 4-ounce serving
Fatty hamburger	lean burger	95 per serving
Pork chop	veal chop	155 per 3-ounce serving
Pork sausage	lean ham	205 per 3-ounce serving
Fried potato	baked	380 per potato
Salad dressing	low-calorie type	65 per tablespoon
Baked beans	green beans	145 per 4-ounce serving
Corn	cauliflower	80 per 4-ounce serving
Club sandwich	bacon, lettuce, and tomato sandwich	175
1 ounce peanuts	1 apple	70

Instead Of	Try This	And Save This Many Calories
1 ounce peanuts	1 ounce grapes	165
1 ounce chocolate	10 pretzels	110

These calorie figures were adapted from *Are You Really Serious About Losing Weight?*, 8th ed. (Philadelphia: Pennwalt, 1975).

These are only a few examples of how you can eat as much food as you do now *and still lose weight*. Think of that: You don't have to eat any less food than you do right now, *but you can still lose weight!*

Even this partial list should show you three or four food servings you could change each day to cut a total of 500 calories. Even if that were the only change you made in your diet, you could thereby *lose one pound* a week, *four pounds* a month, *fifty-two pounds a year!*

That's not such a big change in your diet, and yet even that much would put you in control of your weight. It would let you reduce down to the level you want. And it would reduce your intake of fat and your chances of developing all the problems that excess dietary fat can cause.

But there is even more exciting news ahead. You can tremendously accelerate the weight loss process *and* develop even healthier eating and behavior habits after you read the chapters coming up. (*Caution:* If you take this too fast or too far, you will start knocking against serious hunger. That usually leads to binge eating. Instead, listen to your body and go at the pace that is right for you. Remember, it's not how you start but how you finish the race that counts.)

TO LOSE
BODY FAT
EAT LESS
DIETARY FAT

7

Avoid Excess Sugar

If there's anything that scares dieters, it's those three words, "Avoid excess sugar." The idea in many fad diets that you should give up all sweet treats and desserts is one of the reasons for the downfall of those fad diets. You give up what you like for only so long, and then when you can't take the frustration anymore, you binge on your forbidden treats. The good news in the GIO-KIO diet is that you *don't give up all your favorite sweets.*

Rachel, who is thirty-one and married, said the hardest thing about her old fad diets was "skipping desserts and not feeling full." She said she felt "fatigue and dizziness . . . some people hassled me about not eating at parties." When Rachel crashed off this severe diet, she went on a wild splurge of eating and gained fifteen pounds in just two weeks! But once she got herself on a more sensible diet, she lost twenty-seven pounds in six months. And she has kept it off for a year.

I don't know about you, but I've always had a sweet tooth. I like candy, ice cream, jelly, and other sweet things. Studies of early infant development show that most babies instinctively go for sweet tastes right off the bat. They don't have to learn to like sweets because they're born that way.

93

That means God put those sweet teeth in our heads. He created an amazing number of different sweet sugars in food. We have fructose in raisins and honey, for example; we have sucrose in sugar beets and sugarcane. Milk and milk products contain lactose. Even cereal grains and legumes contain a bit of maltose.

All these chemicals ending in "-ose" are various types of sugar. God created a wide variety of pure, natural, sweet-tasting sugars, and He created our taste receptors for sweetness so that we could appreciate them. So we shouldn't feel guilty about enjoying sweets.

Ah, but there is another side of the story. As with fat, food manufacturers early on discovered that *adding extra sugar* to all sorts of products could make them sell better. God put the sugar in a fresh, wholesome apple. But people mask the natural flavors of other foods by drowning them in sugar in an incredible array of products (e.g., salad dressing, cereals, potato patties). These foods *don't* need sugar in most cases. Sugar is added to make people like them more and buy them more.

Sometimes you have to know the code words for sugar to realize what the food label says. In addition to the sugars already mentioned, you might see words like glucose, dextrose, sorbitol, mannitol, molasses, or maple syrup. These are all sugars. One of my favorite code words is "corn syrup." At first that sounds like some sort of vegetable oil, but it's really a sugary syrup.

The ingredient labels on the products you buy will often list several different added sugars for the same product. In such cases the order of the ingredients listed tells you which is more plentiful in that food item. The list starts with the most plentiful and works its way down to the lesser ones. If one or more sugars are ranked high on the list, that means they are among the most plentiful ingredients in that product.

Start looking at the food labels on the processed foods you eat. You'll find sugar in all kinds of things that you wouldn't normally think needed sugar (e.g., beans, canned spaghetti, seafood casseroles).

Myths About Sugar

1. *It doesn't matter how much sugar you eat as long as you don't gain weight.* False. One of the main problems with a high-sugar diet is that the sweet products displace more healthy, nutritious items. Pure sugar gives you about 113 calories per ounce. This is exactly the same as for protein. If you're giving up protein (or some other nutrient) to make room for extra sugar, you're robbing your own body of what it needs. It's okay to have some sugar in your diet, but avoid so much that you're cutting down on other valuable things.

2. *Eating raisins and other dried fruits with natural sugar is less harmful to your teeth than drinking beverages with added sugar.* False. The type of sugar makes no difference to the teeth. What counts is how long the sugar stays in contact with teeth surfaces. Generally, beverage sugar washes on down. But sugar in sticky foods—either natural ones like raisins or manufactured ones like chewy caramels—tends to hang around the teeth and do more damage. (A neat trick to protect your teeth is to eat some nuts or a raw vegetable immediately after consuming sticky foods with sugar. That helps clean the sticky sweet right off. Brushing the teeth immediately afterward helps even more.)

3. *Regular cola drinks contain only about one or two teaspoons of sugar.* False. They contain about nine teaspoons of sugar. That's a lot more than you would normally add to coffee or tea or some other homemade drink. Of course, sugar-free colas use artificial sweeteners and save about 160 calories per can.

4. *The total amount of sugar added to the typical American diet has declined in recent years.* False. Many people are wising up to the sugar problem and add less by the spoonful from the sugar bowl. But the use of the wide variety of sugars in our food supply has increased. For instance, one study revealed that between 1909

and 1980, the use of all sugars in the food supply
increased by 50 percent![1] Between 1972 and 1980 the
annual use of high-fructose corn syrup alone went up
from two to twenty-six pounds *per person*. No one
adds this syrup at the table; the food companies put it
into the products you buy. Most consumers remain
unaware of this increase in the use of sweets because
they don't know all the words for sugar on food labels.

5. *If you eat a lot of sugar you will grow obese.* That's
only partially true. It's the total calories you eat that
counts, not the type. You could grow fat from too much
sugar. But, ounce for ounce, dietary fat contains more
than twice the calories of sugar. Eating extra fat is more
likely to make you fat than eating extra sugar. However,
excess sugar has other hazards.

6. *Food manufacturers conceal their many uses of sugar
by not mentioning them on the label.* False. In almost
all cases every sugar used is listed on the ingredients
label. However, most consumers don't know all the
words for the various types of sugar. They remain
unaware which products contain sugar, but this is a
question of education rather than deceit by manufacturers.

7. *Foods must have added sugar to maintain their taste
and quality.* False. Some foods that are meant to have
a sweet taste—for example, pie and ice cream—must
have added sugar or other sweeteners. But there is no
reason for adding sugar to cereals, canned spaghetti,
and so on, except increased appeal. When practically
every food has extra sugar to increase appeal, that's too
much. Excess sugar tends to mask natural tastes and
thus reduces the natural variety of flavors in the diet. I
gave up both sugary cereals and adding sugar to plain
cereals years ago, and I've never missed it once since
then.

8. *Raw sugars like honey and brown sugar are more
nutritious than refined table sugars.* Not really. Raw
sugars do contain detectable quantities of some vita-

mins and minerals, but the amounts are not large enough to get excited about.

9. *Maybe natural sugars in excess can be bad for you, but artificial sweeteners can be downright deadly.* This is a common misconception, but a greatly exaggerated one. The Food and Drug Administration (FDA) monitors the safety of artificial sweeteners as well as other food additives. For instance, after nearly two decades of use, cyclamates were banned in this country in 1970. This occurred because of some laboratory evidence that cyclamates might cause cancer in rats consuming huge quantities. If there is any danger to humans, however, it is slight, for cyclamates are still used in Canada without any obvious public health consequences.

The newest popular sweetener is aspartame, and some people are worried about it. But exhaustive research has failed to find any consistent dangers with its use, especially if it is consumed in ordinary quantities.[2] (If you consume too much of anything, including vitamins, you can get sick.)

The latest controversy over artificial sweeteners concerns whether, overall, their use in drinks helps you lose weight or actually makes you gain. It might seem obvious that a drink with only one or two calories couldn't make you gain any weight by itself. But there is a question whether such drinks stimulate your appetite and make you eat more food throughout the day. The issue was brought to light at the 1987 Boston conference of the North American Association for the Study of Obesity, which I was fortunate enough to attend.

Scientists like Robin Kanarek of Tufts University maintain that laboratory animals using artificial sweeteners such as saccharin eat more food and gain more weight than animals drinking only water. However, others like H. S. Koopmans of the University of Calgary point out that animals eating high-calorie sugar drinks gain even more weight.

Apparently, then, drinking sweet drinks carries a double risk for body weight. First, the actual calories in the beverage can be turned into fat and increase the weight problem. That problem

with sugary drinks can be overcome by using low-calorie
artificial sweeteners. However, the second problem is that the
sweet taste of a beverage stimulates the appetite and leads to
greater than normal eating. The conclusion: Drink water, or at
least unsweetened, low-calorie beverages, whenever possible.

What the Bible Says

Refined sugars didn't exist, of course, in Bible times. But
natural sugars like honey were widely prized. As we saw
earlier, in the exodus from Egypt the Israelites were promised
entry into a land "flowing with milk and honey" (Exodus 3:8).
Sweet honey was a symbol of something desirable, something
wonderful.

The Bible clearly recognizes that sugar is also a ready source
of energy. Do you remember when the Israelites under King
Saul were battling the Philistines? Saul had told the soldiers
not to eat before evening came so that they wouldn't stop
pressing the pursuit of their enemies for a moment. Saul's son
Jonathan had not heard this command, so when he got hungry
he stopped to eat some honey: ". . . [he] put his hand to his
mouth; and his eyes became bright" (1 Samuel 14:27). In other
words the sugary energy restored his strength. It made him
vigorous and peppy again. The soldiers who were afraid to eat,
on the other hand, still felt faint. Even though they saved time
by not stopping to eat, they felt so weak that they secured a
lesser victory than if they had been stronger.

There are many meanings in this passage for us today. One is
that honey (and presumably other sugary, high-energy foods)
can restore your strength and help you go about the Lord's
business. Another is that it is foolish to prevent yourself from
eating when you are feeling weak from hunger if you have some
work to do that requires energy. (We'll talk about fasting and
prayer later; that's different.) I know many people who go on
such severe fad diets that they feel too weak to do their jobs.
That's not right. If you need energy, you need energy. Don't diet
so strictly that you interfere with doing God's work.

If eating too little lies at one extreme, eating too much stands at the other. Proverbs 25:27 says, "It is not good to eat much honey." Verse 16 adds, "If you have found honey, eat only enough for you, lest you be sated with it and vomit it."

To sum up, God created sweets and our appreciation of them. He made sugar a good source of energy if eaten in the proper amount. We should neither avoid all sweets nor eat too many sugary foods. The Bible has told us for thousands of years that excess sweets are unhealthy, but only recently has modern science discovered how hazardous an excess it can be.

Health Hazards of Too Much Sugar

The most obvious risk is to your teeth. Sugar in contact with the teeth provides food to the bacteria in your mouth. These bacteria produce acid that eats away at the enamel on your teeth. In time tooth decay sets in and you need to go to a dentist to get drilled and filled.

I remember many times sitting uncomfortably in a dentist's chair wondering how on earth people 500 or 2500 years ago could survive tooth decay and rot without dentists. I recently learned the answer from Dr. James Shaw of the Harvard School of Dental Medicine. It seems that in ancient times they had less tooth decay than now. God designed teeth to last a lifetime, and until the invention of refined sugars and their spread throughout the food supply, teeth usually did last a lifetime. Examination of skulls reveals that prehistoric men often had better teeth than children of modern times.

One of the worst things a parent can do is to give bottles of sweetened juice to babies in the crib as they're falling asleep. This steady contact with sugar, if it recurs often over a few months, can rot a baby's new teeth. You see, it's the length of time that sugar touches the teeth that counts. A little sugar during meals won't hurt much. But a continuous sipping on sugary drinks or chewing on candy throughout the day can cause serious damage.

Adult diabetes represents another health hazard. There is some controversy, however, because the exact causes of adult diabetes mellitus are not entirely known. We do know, however, that to metabolize or use sugar you need the hormone insulin. Diabetics of this type produce plenty of insulin, but for some reason their bodies don't respond to it properly. Their blood sugar rises since they can't take it out of the blood and use it in their bodily cells at the proper rate. It's sort of like a leaky boat. If your bilge pump (insulin) works well, you can keep the bilge water level (blood sugar) down. But if your pump slows down, the water level in your boat rises. Until we learn definitely otherwise, I think it's safe to suspect that excess sugar either helps cause diabetes, or at least makes it worse. Eating too much sugar is like punching holes in your boat to let in more water.

As we've seen, an excess of *any* nutrient can help add to the body fat problem. Sugar contains as many calories per ounce as protein, namely, 113. If you ate thirty-one ounces of sugar (in the form of candy and other sweets) and didn't burn off any of the resulting 3500 calories, your body would turn the excess calories into another pound of body fat. Furthermore, sugar in the diet tends to increase the appetite and encourages you to eat more calories in general, according to Dr. Paula J. Geiselman of the University of California at Los Angeles. This is not simply a matter of self-deception: Biochemical processes in the body are stimulated by sugar.

Dr. Kenneth C. Hayes of Brandeis University has investigated heart disease and sugar. Although the explanation is complex, the conclusion of the study is this: If animal fats and cholesterol pose a double whammy for the heart, adding excess sugar to the picture makes it into a triple whammy. Your heart and excess sugar don't get along.

Is sugar addictive? Because some people eat sugar at every opportunity, some commentators have likened sugar craving to a sort of drug addiction. But experts on addiction are quick to point out the differences between this kind of craving and true addiction.[3] The essence of addiction is avoiding the painful state known as *withdrawal* when one stops taking a certain kind of drug. But people flock to sugar because of the pleasure it provides, not to avoid a painful state caused by its absence. The absence of sugar might make one long for it again, but does not cause genuine physical pain in the sense that withdrawal from alcohol or heroin does. In short, sugar craving may become a powerful habit, but it is not a true addiction.

Do You Eat Too Much Sugar?

Take the following little quiz and let's find out. Circle the letter of your answer according to the following scale:

A = less than once a week, or never
B = once or twice a week
C = three to five times a week
D = daily or almost daily

How often do you do the following:

1. Drink sweetened drinks, for example, canned or bottled colas and fruit drinks? (Don't count sugar-free drinks sweetened with aspartame or another artificial sweetener.)   A B C D
2. Eat sweet desserts or snacks such as pastries and ice cream?   A B C D
3. Use fruits commercially packed in sugar syrup or add sugar to fruit at the table?   A B C D
4. Eat candy?   A B C D
5. Add sugar to coffee, tea, or other drinks?   A B C D
6. Use jam, jelly, honey, or other natural sweeteners?   A B C D

Adapted from *Dietary Guidelines for Americans*, U. S. Department of Agriculture: Home and Garden Bulletin Number 232–5 (April, 1986), p. 4.

Anything you circled in the first two columns is fine. Remember, a little sugar in your diet is okay. It makes eating more enjoyable. If you have more than three marks in the third column, you should consider cutting down. We're going to see what you can do about replacing these items with others that *also* taste sweet, but are much better for you. If you have any marks in the last column, consider how you might be able to reduce your intake of refined sugars. It's not worth the risk to your health, particularly since there are so many other fine foods that you can substitute.

Guidelines for Cutting Down on Sugar

1. If you have any doubt about which food products contain sugar, always read the ingredients label before purchasing. Remember the different words for sugar: Most end in -ose (e.g., sucrose, glucose, galactose, fructose) or -tol (e.g., sorbitol, mannitol); others are called "syrup," including corn syrup, maple syrup, and so on. If you like the item, go ahead and buy it. Remember, a little sugar is okay, as long as you know what you're eating. But if you suddenly realize that what you're about to buy has three different added sugars and you don't want to get your sugar in that form, then *don't* buy it. As Isaiah 55:2 says, "Why do you spend your money for that which is not bread, and your labor for that which does not satisfy? Hearken diligently to me, and eat what is good. . . ."

2. All fruits already contain the sugars that God put in to start with. In general buy and eat fruits fresh or packed in water and avoid canned fruits packed in sweet syrup.

3. Try to minimize the use of foods loaded in refined sugars: candies, jams, jellies, syrups, and sugary drinks. If you like these things, consume some but cut down the amounts.

4. Reduce the amount of sugar you use in recipes for home-cooked foods. You might find that you can reduce the sugar load by 25 or 50 percent or more and not miss it at all! Too much sugar overwhelms the natural flavors of the other ingredients. Paradoxically, less sugar sometimes tastes better. Experiment until you find the balance that is right for you and your family.

5. Instead of relying on sugar all the time, accentuate the flavors of foods with spices. This allows you to enhance the natural taste, if you wish, but also to experience a more lively variety in your diet. It also cuts down on calories. For instance, in a recipe for apple pie try cutting out half the sugar but adding cinnamon to improve the flavor. Other handy spices to keep around the house are cardamom, coriander, nutmeg, ginger, and mace.

6. Depending on your schedule and how much you like to cook, try using fewer commercially prepared items like baked goods, canned spaghetti, and soups. Create your own from scratch. This gives you greater knowledge of *what* is going into the recipe and of *how much*.

7. Save sweet foods like baked goods, candy, and ice cream for desserts rather than snacks. On an empty stomach you might eat too much of these high-calorie goodies. But on a full stomach, only a little might satisfy you as much. You'll be happier when you look at the bathroom scale the next morning.

8. For snacks and many of your desserts reach for foods like fruit that have natural sweeteners. Try to cut down on foods with lots of sugars packed in during processing.

9. At the table try to minimize use of the sugar bowl. (I don't even keep one on the table anymore.) For coffee and tea use artificial sweeteners like aspartame that are almost calorie-free. If you must add sugar to drinks, cereal, and so on, start cutting back gradually. You might find, as I did, that many foods taste better *without* added sugar.

10. Reduce the number of drinks with sugar that you consume: sweetened fruit drinks, punches, and ades. Drink water to satisfy thirst whenever possible. If you like carbonated drinks, juices, and punches, go for the low-cal ones without added sugar.

These guidelines and the myths about sugar were adapted in
part from material in *Dietary Guidelines for Americans*, U. S.
Department of Agriculture: Home and Garden Bulletin Number
232–5 (April, 1986).

Reducing Sugar Intake *Works*

These guidelines work. Ginger is thirty-three years old and
recently had her second child. She has tried some of the popular
fad diets and says, "I got frustrated with them if I didn't lose
weight fast. I got bored and discouraged because it was so slow."
She explained that her greatest problem in living on these diets
was giving up *all* her favorite sweets. "Ice cream and chocolate
are my passions," she says.

That is one of the classic mistakes in fad diets: You give up
all the foods you like and suffer through foods you don't like.
With the GIO-KIO diet and health plan you *don't have to give
up all your desserts,* just cut down on the ones with huge
amounts of added sugar and added fat. Then practice food
substitution wherever possible. Learn to appreciate the foods
that are naturally sweet as God designed them.

Once she got her act together, Ginger lost thirty-four pounds
in just six months, declining from 158 to 124. Now she
says,"My husband's reaction to my thinner self was encourag-
ing!" About dieting she says, "Stay on it; it feels so much better
in every way to be thin."

Elizabeth had a somewhat similar problem due to a diet
plan that kept her away from all desserts. At thirty-one,
married, with a new job as a family nurse practitioner, she
didn't have a lot of weight she needed to lose. She only
weighed 120 pounds. She sounds like Ginger when she
complains about her old diet: "I get depressed if I know I can't
have dessert. I love ice cream and enjoy snacks at night. That's
probably my worst time."

Elizabeth is right that eating sweet desserts as snacks just
before bedtime is not a good idea. That gives you less chance to
burn off the calories. If you lie there asleep while digesting the
sweets, the excess calories are likely to start turning into fat

before you wake up. On the other hand, don't deprive yourself of some sweets at your regular mealtime. Once Elizabeth got over her mental block, she lost six pounds and reached her ideal weight of 114.

I think it is somewhat amazing that only in the last few years have the United States Department of Agriculture and the Human Nutrition Information Service published *Dietary Guidelines for Americans*. One of these guidelines states, "Avoid too much sugar." It took hundreds of years for modern governments to recognize the importance of that concept to public health. Yet the Bible told us that thousands of years ago.

ENJOY FOODS
THAT ARE SWEET
AS GOD MADE THEM

8

Avoid Excess Protein

I remember as a kid reading about athletes who ate only high-protein foods like steak. The idea was that if muscles are made of protein, and you want to build muscle, you must eat only protein. Wrong!

You certainly do want to eat plenty of balanced protein. Too little *is* dangerous. But treating your body as if it were one large muscle that only needs protein is a little crazy, to say the least. Different parts of your body have different requirements. The brain, for example, needs protein to form its cells, but it normally uses glucose (sugar) for energy. Also, excess protein is bad for other organ systems, as we'll see later. Many fad diets stress either too much or too little protein. Either extreme can have unpleasant consequences.

What *Is* Protein?

A protein is made up of a sequence of amino acids, or types of chemical molecules. There are about twenty amino acids, and they can be arranged in different sequences to form different proteins. It is similar to the twenty-six letters of the alphabet, which can be arranged in different ways to form an almost infinite variety of words.

Of these amino acids, eight are essential and twelve are nonessential. Essential acids are those the human body can't produce, so they *must* come from the diet. Therefore, if you don't eat balanced protein that contains these eight, you will in time pay the price.

The nonessential amino acids can be produced in the body, but not from thin air. Usually the body takes one amino acid in plentiful supply and transforms it into one that is needed. For these nonessential amino acids the balance of the protein doesn't matter so much, but the total amount does.

Think of your protein intake as financial income. If you have plenty available, you can make change. You can convert two five-dollar bills into a ten, for instance. But if you're short of total cash, you can't make change. So even the nonessential amino acids are "essential" in the sense that you need them. You must derive them either directly from food or from other amino acids derived from food. Either way, a good diet is still the key to providing the right amount of protein.

Uses of Protein

Protein is a vital nutrient for the following reasons:

- All living cells require protein, so you must consume enough for growth and replacement of dead cells.
- Many hormones, those chemicals that control bodily functions like growth and sexual development, depend on protein.
- All enzymes, those molecules that control thousands of different chemical reactions in the body, are composed of protein.
- The immune system requires protein, for instance, to produce antibodies to fight disease.

There are many other uses of protein, but these should show how important this nutrient really is. By contrast, the main bodily use for many sugars is as energy. Proteins can even take the place of that, since they can be converted into energy, too.

Health Hazards of Excess Protein

Protein is absolutely essential for life, but an excess does carry a risk.

Too much of any calorie-containing nutrient helps contribute to obesity. Protein contains as many calories as sugar and other carbohydrates. However, dietary protein is probably less dangerous than fat or sugar because it tends to squelch the appetite quicker. On the other hand, most high-protein foods like meat and cheese are also high in fat. So when you eat too much protein, you usually eat too much fat as well.

We think of a thick, juicy sirloin steak as mostly protein. While it does contain plenty of high-quality protein, about 56 percent of its calories are due to fat. Careful trimming of all visible fat still leaves the steak with about 36 percent of its calories in fat. Remember, most fat in food is not clearly visible.

The kidneys and liver, important in handling the body's load of ingested protein, can be strained by too much of this nutrient.[1] Excess protein makes them work too hard and can cause damage. Also, elimination of the metabolic waste from protein requires the kidneys to use up a lot of water. This can have a dehydrating effect on the body. Excess protein also causes the kidneys to lose too much of the body's precious supply of calcium (needed for strong bones and teeth).

High-protein diets do tend to subdue the appetite, hence their popularity. But eating too much protein tends to displace from the diet other valuable foods like grains, vegetables, and fruit. These others are needed, too, to maintain balance. Without the fiber they provide, constipation becomes common.

Finally, fad diets high in protein and fat, thus low in important carbohydrates, tend to make people feel tired, nervous, and apathetic.

What the Bible Says

The Israelites wandering in the wilderness were not a happy
lot. Do you remember when God gave them manna from heaven
to eat? We use the phrase "manna from heaven" to symbolize
God's special providence and blessing. But how did the people
who actually ate it day after day react? Were they grateful to
God for His blessing? No! They complained!

Here they were, gathering food for which they had neither
tilled the ground nor sown. God provided it free. Instead of
rejoicing and praising God, they moaned about all the wonderful meat in Egypt that they had left behind. They said, "Would
that we had died by the Lord's hand in the land of Egypt, when
we sat by the pots of meat, when we ate bread to the full; for you
have brought us out into this wilderness to kill this whole
assembly with hunger" (Exodus 16:3 NAS).

Doesn't that sound like a typical dieter's lament? He misses
all those juicy pork chops, sirloin steaks, and dripping cheeseburgers. He used to chow down all he wanted. Now he feels
like he's about to starve on a more simple diet. But he won't
starve on a balanced diet any more than the Israelites starved in
the wilderness.

According to Numbers 11, the Israelites kept complaining
until Moses couldn't stand it anymore. He said he would rather
die than listen to the people complain about the lack of meat
(vv. 13–15). God gave them meat, but in a punishing way. He
said they would eat quail "until it comes out of your nostrils
and you loathe it" (v. 20). And as they gathered the meat and
began their feast, God struck them with a plague (v. 33).

That sounds a bit like a fad dieter who's been so deprived
that he goes on a binge. He eats huge quantities of the very thing
he's been depriving himself of, but then he pays the price for
his gorging by getting sick.

In addition to teaching us about trust in God and other moral
lessons, these passages also teach a dietary lesson. Excess meat
protein simply isn't good for us. And because we might crave it
doesn't mean that we need it. If we eat too much, we will pay
the price.

Health Hazards of Too Little Protein

Having too little protein is probably the most common nutritional problem in the world. In lands where there is famine and people are dying of starvation, protein deficiency is the key cause.

In modern industrialized societies such terrible poverty is thankfully rare. Protein deficiency usually occurs only as a result of fad dieting. There may also be protein imbalance in the diet. Some of the consequences are the following:

- *Muscle wasting.* Think of your muscles in part as storage bins for protein. Your body must have protein every day. If you don't eat any or don't eat enough, your body will take from the store in your muscles. Since you don't really have extra in your muscles, this means that your muscles will begin to waste away. You will literally make yourself weaker. Extreme fad diets with insufficient protein have actually killed people, in part because muscles like the heart grow so weak that they can't sustain life.[2]
- *Stunting of growth.* The body must have protein to grow. An insufficient amount during childhood and adolescence can cause permanent stunting of growth and development. This is the main reason that young people should never diet except when under the care of a physician.
- *Resistance to disease.* The immune system is weakened by a lack of protein, so the person is more likely to fall prey to any of the disease organisms that are circulating in his region of the country.
- *Other physical symptoms.* Not everyone on a low-protein diet gets all the following symptoms. But everyone gets some of these or related problems if she sticks with insufficient protein too long: decreased blood pressure, decreased body temperature, bloating, hair loss, diarrhea, or gout. Remember, every bodily system requires protein in some way, and insufficient protein can affect practically every system eventually. This bloating, by the way, can paradoxically make the person look fat. But in

this case, the bulging, ballooning effect is due not to fat but to excess fluid trapped in the tissues by the lack of protein.

Guidelines for Protein Consumption

1. Because some amino acids are essential while others are not, and because food proteins vary so much in composition, it is important to get a balance of protein. In other words, if you were to eat nothing but rice, your diet would get plenty of some amino acids, but remain lacking in others. Generally speaking, if you eat meat and other animal products as well as vegetable products, you will get enough balance in your protein.

2. Vegetarians, on the other hand, must eat special combinations of plant foods to get the right mix. For instance, beans provide one mix of amino acids, while grains provide another. Either category by itself is insufficient, but together they provide the right mix. We call such foods as the following *complementary proteins:*

> beans and rice
> beans and corn
> nuts and vegetables
> peanut butter and bread
> macaroni and cheese

This last example goes beyond strict vegetarianism to include animal milk products (cheese). You can use these vegetarian combinations to cut down on your intake of animal protein (and its associated fat and cholesterol) and yet still get balanced, high-quality protein.

3. Foods high in protein include meat, poultry, and fish; milk products like cheese and yogurt; legumes like beans and peas; nuts and eggs. The problem is that most of these foods, with the exception of legumes, also contain quite a bit of fat. Try to use the leanest meat you can find, and the lowest fat milk and yogurt.

Some cheeses can't be made with less fat, so restrict your intake of them. Most cheeses have about 60 to 80 percent of their calories in fat. The same holds for peanuts, cashews, and other nuts. It takes a lot of low-fat foods to make up for foods that high in fat and still get your average down to below 30 percent of your total calories in fat.

4. You do *not* need to eat meat with every meal. But to most Americans, nothing beats a good, thick steak or juicy roast. In truth, there is a lot to be said for lean, red meat. But most people get too much protein in this way and tend to overlook other sources. The typical American diet might include bacon for breakfast (74 percent fat), bologna for lunch (80 percent fat), and ground beef for dinner (66 percent fat). That's too much meat protein *and* too much fat.

5. To figure your exact protein requirement each day, multiply your body weight in pounds times 0.36 grams. For example, a 110-pound woman needs about 40 grams of protein a day (110 × 0.36 grams = 39.6 grams). To see how much food you need to reach that total, see the following chart:[3]

The Amount of Protein in Food

Food	Grams of Protein	Per Serving Size
Meat	7	1 ounce
Vegetables	2	4 ounces
French fries	2	10 strips
Bread	2	1 slice
Cereal	2	1 ounce
Milk products	8	1 cup
Cheese	6	1-ounce slice

The typical fast-food lunch, all by itself, provides more protein than this 110-pound woman needs. Let's add it up:

Quarter-pound burger	=	28 g protein (4 oz. × 7)
One slice of cheese	=	6
Two slices bread	=	4
Vegetable trimmings	=	1
French fries	=	4
Milk shake	=	10
Total:		53 grams of protein

This woman's recommended protein need per day is 40 grams and she gets more than that just for lunch! A little more than the minimum is, of course, all right. But if she eats like that at every meal, she will get three or four times as much protein as she needs. That's way too much.

6. Try to replace some of your red meat intake with fish. Both have plenty of good protein, but fish has something extra—omega-three fish oils—that might improve your health. Dr. K. Frank Austen, a professor of medicine at Harvard Medical School, has demonstrated that these fish oils are great for your heart.[4] When consumed in a regular diet at least three times a week, fish helps to prevent cardiovascular (heart) diseases and also so-called inflammatory diseases like asthma and arthritis.

EAT ENOUGH
PROTEIN
BUT NOT *TOO* MUCH

9

Avoid Excess Salt

In societies where a lot of salt is not added to the food supply, blood pressure changes little with age.[1] But in societies that do add salt, and this includes advanced nations like the United States, blood pressure keeps going up with age. Currently in the United States about one-quarter of the population has significant hypertension (elevated blood pressure).

Hypertension has been called "the silent killer" because you don't feel it, and you remain unaware of it except when blood pressure is measured. Just because you don't know about it does not mean it can't hurt you. Hypertension contributes to heart attacks, strokes, and kidney problems.

In general excess salt seems able to raise blood pressure, often to dangerous levels. Some recent new research has shown that not every individual is sensitive to this salt–blood pressure connection. In other words, *some* people can eat lots of salt and not see their blood pressure go up. But unless you know *for sure* that you fall into the safe group, it would be wiser not to take the chance. If *any* of your blood relatives have high blood pressure, you probably are not in the safe group.

Reduce your salt intake as much as you can, without going so far as to ruin the palatability of your diet. This is not just a matter of deleting the salt shaker from the table. I do recommend that. But as in the case of sugar, more salt is added to the food supply at the manufacturing level than at the table. Many people remain unaware of which and how many foods are steeped in salt *even without adding a single grain at the dining table.*

Do You Get Too Much Salt?

Take this little test to find out. As before, circle the letter that indicates how often you eat each of the following, using this scale:

A = less than once a week
B = once or twice a week
C = three to five times a week
D = daily or almost daily

How often do you do the following:

1. Eat cured or processed meats such as ham, bacon, sausage, hot dogs, and lunch meats? A B C D
2. Eat canned or frozen vegetables that include a sauce? A B C D
3. Eat TV dinners, canned soups, or other commercially packaged meals? A B C D
4. Eat cheese? A B C D
5. Eat salted nuts, chips, and other snacks? A B C D
6. Add salt when cooking vegetables, rice, or pasta? A B C D
7. Add salt or other salty condiments like soy sauce, steak sauce, catsup, mustard, salad dressings, or seasoning mixes to your food? A B C D
8. Sprinkle salt on your food even before tasting it? A B C D

This and the Guidelines section on pages 119, 120 were adapted in part from *Dietary Guidelines for Americans,* U. S. Department of Agriculture:Home and Garden Bulletin Number 232–6(April, 1986), pp. 4–6.

How did you do? All eight of these items involve adding salt to your diet. Anything you circled in the first two columns is probably all right. However, I would recommend deleting cured meats (item 1) and salted snacks (item 5) as much as possible. These items not only have loads of salt, but usually lots of fat as well. If you have more than two items in the third column, I hope you'll consider cutting down. If there's anything in the fourth column, I would definitely try to reduce that.

I realize that if you go through a bag of chips a night while watching TV it's going to be difficult to cut down. Any long-established habit will take some time to break. Start by cutting down a little at a time if you have to. If you can, go cold turkey on salty snacks and replace them with healthier food like fresh fruit and vegetables.

Some of the items on the list, as well as providing salt and fat, also provide some good nutrients like protein. Cheese, for instance, is in many ways a wonderful food. By all means, eat some, but don't overdo it. Unfortunately, cheese remains loaded with fat and salt. I adore practically all kinds of cheese, and I know it's difficult to choose less. But try to replace at least some of what you're eating with other dairy products or other foods.

Salt in the Food Supply

You may be wondering why food manufacturers add so much salt. With nuts, popcorn, and chips, it's optional. They add it because many people feel it enhances flavor, but you don't really need it. With sausage or cheese, salt must be added to make the product. If you tried to make cheese without salt and followed every other step but did not add salt, you wouldn't come out with cheese as we know it. In other words, cheese wouldn't be cheese without salt; it is absolutely necessary. Therefore, the only way to cut down is to reduce the amount of those foods that you eat.

As in the case of sugar, the addition of salt to food is

sometimes disguised by the number of different terms that include it on the food label. Actually, the problem is even more complex than for sugar. You see, it's not really salt (or sodium chloride) as a whole that can hurt you. It's just the sodium. So when you see words like *monosodium glutamate* and *sodium citrate* on the food label, that's just as bad as salt, garlic salt, onion salt, and so on. Watch out for products with lots of sodium-containing ingredients on the label.

Sodium can hurt you because after you eat it, it gets into the blood. There, it can only be chemically balanced by pulling more water into the blood. Salty snacks make you thirsty because, in a sense, they dehydrate the body. Furthermore, the excess water in the blood can make the blood pressure rise. It's like turning the faucet way up when you're watering the lawn. With more water running through the hose, you can literally feel the pressure inside the tube as you hold it.

Guidelines for Reducing Excess Salt

Except for people with rare diseases who can't retain a normal salt balance in the body, virtually everyone gets more salt than they need. Salt is an essential nutrient, but you can get more than enough by eating plain, unprocessed foods. Fresh, uncooked, untreated fruits and vegetables and meats already contain plenty. Salt was built in during the growth of the organism. Thus there is no reason to worry about a deficiency; in fact most people get twenty to thirty times as much as they need.

Here are some suggestions on how to reduce the sodium in your diet:

1. Read the labels on the foods you buy. If you see lots of sodium-containing ingredients, think of an alternative item you can buy instead.
2. Buy fresh, unprocessed items and prepare them your-

self, whenever possible. Most processed and convenience foods have loads of sodium.

3. Look for the newly developed and marketed products that are unusually low in sodium. *One caution:* Salt is added, in part, as a food preservative. Low-sodium foods, therefore, don't last as long in storage as others. For instance, low-salt lunch meats will turn bad faster than regular ones, so eat these items promptly.

4. Add as little sodium as you feel comfortable with when cooking. Recognize, however, that certain items like baked goods *require* some sodium or they can't be made.

5. Try to replace sodium as a seasoning and flavoring agent with one of the new potassium chloride salt replacers or with herbs and spices (more on this in the next section). But beware of using condiments like mustard and catsup as an alternative to sodium. They contain salt, too.

6. Get rid of the salt shaker at the table. If your food needs extra seasoning, add an herb blend. You can buy a blend or make your own, fill a shaker with it, and sprinkle it on instead of salt. Here are three recipes for such herb blends:

Herb Blends to Replace Salt

Saltless surprise:
2 teaspoons garlic powder and 1 teaspoon each of basil, oregano, and powdered lemon rind (or dehydrated lemon juice). Put ingredients into a blender and mix well. Store in glass container, label well, and add rice to prevent caking.

Pungent salt substitute:
3 teaspoons basil, 2 teaspoons each of savory (summer savory is best), celery seed, ground cumin seed, sage, and marjoram, and 1 teaspoon lemon thyme. Mix well, then powder with a mortar and pestle.

Spicy *saltless* seasoning:
1 teaspoon each of cloves,
pepper, and coriander seed
(crushed), 2 teaspoons paprika, and 1 tablespoon
rosemary. Mix ingredients
in a blender. Store in air-
tight container.

Source: "Do Yourself a Flavor," *FDA Consumer* (April, 1984),
Department of Health and Human Services Publication No.
(FDA) 84–2192, p. 4.

You may find that some items don't taste good without salt.
Okay. If you don't have hypertension, go ahead and add a little
salt. But try to get by with the least you need. I can do without
added salt in practically every food except popcorn. To me,
popcorn isn't popcorn without salt.

On the other hand, as you reduce salt you may find that some
foods actually taste better that way. Salt can be a flavor
enhancer, but it can also be a flavor masker. The more you use
it, the more alike different foods taste. As you reduce salt, you
can begin to recognize—and *enjoy*—a host of flavors that you
never even realized were there before.

Using Herbs and Spices

Many people rely mostly on sugar and salt to flavor foods.
They remain largely unaware of the rich variety of herbs and
spices that God created. For instance, Exodus 30:23–24
mentions myrrh, cinnamon, fragrant cane, and cassia. (Some
of these were used in incense or ointments rather than food.)
Numbers 11:5–6 mentions leeks, onions, and garlic, and how
such seasoners increase appetite. Matthew 13:31 mentions
mustard, and Matthew 23:23 mentions that the Pharisees
even tithed (inappropriately) such spices as mint, dill, and
cumin.

Different combinations of herbs and spices can introduce you
to delicious dishes you have never known before. Here are a
few suggestions as to which of these seasoning agents go with
which foods:

What Goes With What

Soups	Bay, chervil, French tarragon, marjoram, parsley, savory, rosemary
Poultry	Garlic, oregano, rosemary, savory, sage
Beef	Bay, chives, cloves, cumin, garlic, hot pepper, marjoram, rosemary, savory
Lamb	Garlic, marjoram, oregano, rosemary, thyme (make little slits in lamb to be roasted and insert herbs)
Pork	Coriander, cumin, garlic, ginger, hot pepper, pepper sage, savory, thyme
Cheese	Basil, chervil, chives, curry, dill, fennel, garlic chives, marjoram, oregano, parsley, sage, thyme
Fish	Chervil, dill, fennel, French tarragon, garlic, parsley, thyme
Fruit	Anise, cinnamon, coriander, cloves, ginger, lemon verbena, mint, rose geranium, sweet cicely
Bread	Caraway, marjoram, oregano, poppy seed, rosemary, thyme
Vegetables	Basil, burnet, chervil, chives, dill, French tarragon, marjoram, mint, parsley, pepper, thyme
Salads	Basil, borage, burnet, chives, parsley, rocket-salad, sorrel (these are best used fresh or added to salad dressing—otherwise, use herb vinegars for extra flavor)

Source: "Do Yourself a Flavor," *FDA Consumer* (April, 1984), Department of Health and Human Services Publication No. (FDA) 84–2192, p. 4.

SPICES AND HERBS

Vegetable	Spices or herbs
Asparagus	Mustard seed, sesame seed, or tarragon
Lima beans	Marjoram, oregano, sage, savory, tarragon, or thyme
Snap beans	Basil, dill, marjoram, mint, mustard seed, oregano, savory, tarragon, or thyme
Beets	Allspice, bay leaves, caraway seed, cloves, dill, ginger, mustard seed, savory, or thyme
Broccoli	Caraway seed, dill, mustard seed, or tarragon
Brussels sprouts	Basil, caraway seed, dill, mustard seed, sage, or thyme
Cabbage	Caraway seed, celery seed, dill, mint, mustard seed, nutmeg, savory, or tarragon
Carrots	Allspice, bay leaves, caraway seed, dill, fennel, ginger, mace, marjoram, mint, nutmeg, or thyme
Cauliflower	Caraway seed, celery salt, dill, mace, or tarragon
Cucumbers	Basil, dill, mint, or tarragon
Eggplant	Marjoram or oregano
Onions	Caraway seed, mustard seed, nutmeg, oregano, sage, or thyme
Peas	Basil, dill, marjoram, mint, oregano, poppy seed, rosemary, sage, or savory
Potatoes	Basil, bay leaves, caraway seed, celery seed, dill, chives, mustard seed, oregano, poppy seed, or thyme
Spinach	Basil, mace, marjoram, nutmeg, or oregano
Squash	Allspice, basil, cinnamon, cloves, fennel, ginger, mustard seed, nutmeg, or rosemary
Sweet potatoes	Allspice, cardamom, cinnamon, cloves, or nutmeg
Tomatoes	Basil, bay leaves, celery seed, oregano, sage, sesame seed, tarragon, or thyme
Green salads	Basil, chives, dill, or tarragon

Source: Vegetables in Family Meals, U. S. Deparment of Agriculture: Home and Garden Bulletin No. 105 (1968), p. 18.

Next time you go to the grocery store, I recommend you buy some herbs and spices you've never had before. Bring them home and experiment. You can use them to reduce your reliance on salt, sugar, and fat, and you will open yourself up to the adventure of enjoying new and different dishes.

LESS SALT =
LESS HEALTH RISK

10

The Need for Carbohydrates

In previous chapters we looked at cutting down on fat, sweets, protein, and total calories. But here is one nutrient that most people need to *increase* in their diets. Aren't you glad there is at least one you can increase and enjoy more, and still lose weight? With this diet plan you need not restrict yourself to tiny portions of everything. If you choose foods wisely, you can eat more, not less than you do now, and *still* lose weight!

We must make an important distinction between the two major types of carbohydrates. There are *complex carbohydrates*, mainly the vegetable starches, and *simple carbohydrates*, or the sugars. Because most people get too much sugar, except possibly for the kinds found in fruit (we covered sweets in chapter 7), we are talking mostly about complex carbohydrates, about starch and fiber.

Let's see if you are getting enough complex carbohydrates. As before, indicate the frequency with which you eat each food by circling the most accurate letter, according to the following scale:

A = rarely or never
B = once or twice a week
C = three or four times a week
D = daily or almost daily

How often do you eat:

1. Several servings of grain foods like bread,
   cereal, or pasta?   A B C D
2. Whole-grain breads or cereals?   A B C D
3. Starchy vegetables like potatoes, corn,
   beans, and peas?   A B C D
4. Several servings of vegetables?   A B C D
5. Several servings of fresh fruit?   A B C D

Adapted from *Dietary Guidelines for Americans*, U.S. Department of Agriculture: Home and Garden Bulletin Number 232–4 (April, 1986), p. 1.

The best answer for all five of these questions is "almost daily" (D). If you circled anything else, consider what you've been missing in your diet and think about adding more. You will stave off the munchies as you cut down on sugar and fat.

Let's take a closer look at these kinds of foods:

1. *Grain products.* Many fad diets want you to cut down on these, but that's not a good idea. Grain products are not as fattening as most people think, at least not by themselves. It's what you add to them that starts picking up your fat and calorie count. For example, a slice of whole-wheat bread has only seventy calories and one gram of fat. But each pat of butter adds thirty-five calories and four grams of fat. And two tablespoons of jelly adds 100 calories more. So it's not the plain bread that gets you in the tummy department, it's the extras that triple the calories and quadruple the fat. Of course, plain toast is not tasty. I'm not recommending that you do without all condiments but that you cut down wherever possible. You can use margarine instead of butter and save about half the calories and fat. You can cut down on the amount of margarine you add, slowly reducing till you find the least amount that you can still enjoy.

2. *Whole grains.* You should have whole-grain products every day. That's the only kind humans ate for thousands of years. But within the last century food chemists began to study carbohydrates in grains. When they first investigated the bran and the germ in the wheat kernel, they didn't realize the nutrients contained there. They thought they were purifying the food by removing this "unimportant" matter. They thought it was a great achievement to be able to offer refined, white flour that was almost pure carbohydrate, the main wheat nutrient they recognized. They didn't realize (at first) that they had thrown out most of the other nutrients! By the time they did, people had come to prefer lighter flours and breads. So manufacturers began to chemically add back some of the nutrients that they had thrown away by excess milling. But even enriched white bread has less phosphorus, potassium, iron, and fiber than whole-wheat bread. Not only is whole-wheat more nutritious but most people, given a fair amount of exposure to both types, like the taste and mouth-feel of whole-wheat better.

3. *Starchy vegetables.* You need potatoes or other starchy vegetables almost daily. Fad diets may warn you away from starches, and the potato is often taboo. But an entire half-pound potato, if you remove the skin, has only 145 calories and no fat. (The skin adds about 75 calories but no fat.) But two tablespoons of butter adds 200 calories and 22 grams of fat. As with grain products, a potato doesn't taste very good plain. I don't eat it that way, and I'm not suggesting that you do either. But cut down on the extras as much as you can and still maintain your enjoyment. Or practice replacement. For example, two tablespoons of sour cream adds only 50 calories and 6 grams of fat. So you can add the same amount but a different type of condiment and save about three-quarters of the calories and the fat. Trying it different ways at

different times also gives you more variety. (See a recipe for a delicious, low-calorie, low-fat topping in chapter 16.)

4. *Vegetables.* As we've already seen, you should have several servings of vegetables a day. They are a rich source of vitamins and minerals as well as fiber. Eat vegetables fresh whenever possible, either plain as snacks, in salads, or as accompaniments to sandwiches and other dishes. Cooking vegetables destroys some of the nutrients.

5. *Fruit.* You should have several servings of fruit each day as well. This is the best way to get your sweets. Again, eat these fresh and whole whenever possible.

The Value of Dietary Fiber

Fiber is a vegetable or plant material that humans can't digest (although certain other animals can). Chemically, a molecule of either fiber or starch is composed of molecules of sugar. But the human digestive tract simply can't break down fiber as it can the starch in potatoes or pasta.

What this means is that fiber passes all the way through the gastrointestinal tract. As it does, it absorbs water and produces a larger mass in the stool so that this waste is evacuated more quickly and easily. In other words, fiber helps prevent constipation. In fact, fiber seems to be nature's main way of doing that.

In addition, fiber also absorbs some of the fat and cholesterol liberated during digestion. Fiber in your diet is not only calorie-free in itself, it helps snatch extra calories out of your system before you can absorb them. The best fibers for reducing your cholesterol level are those in apples and other fruits, carrots, chick-peas, oats, soybeans, and other beans. Because fiber helps in the elimination of solid waste, it keeps the colon and rectum healthy. There is mounting evidence that fiber may actually reduce the risks of cancers, inflammations, and other diseases at these sites.

Guidelines for Getting the Right Amount of Fiber

The average American eats only about eleven grams of fiber a day. That's not nearly enough and may be one reason for constipation, spastic colon, colon and rectal cancer, hemorrhoids, appendicitis, diverticulosis, and related problems often observed in advanced societies.[1] The National Cancer Institute recommends that we eat about twice that much fiber, or between twenty and thirty grams a day. However, don't think that the more fiber, the better. More than thirty-five grams a day may cause some negative effects. For example, it might cause too much bulk and frequency of stools. If too little fiber leads to constipation, too much can lead to diarrhea.

How can you get the right amount of fiber? Here are some common high-fiber foods:

Food	Grams Fiber	Per Serving Size
All-bran type cereals	8	⅓ cup
Popcorn	2.5	1 cup
Whole-wheat bread	1.4	1 slice
Legumes	4–7	½ cup
Vegetables	1–3	½ cup
Fresh fruit	2–3	1 piece
Dried prunes	1	1 prune

If you eat a variety of foods, as discussed in chapter 5, you will have no trouble reaching an optimum amount of fiber. Imagine getting, as recommended in the GIO-KIO plan, four servings of vegetables (about eight grams of fiber), three servings of fruit (about seven grams), and four slices of whole-wheat bread (about six grams) in one day. That would provide twenty-one grams of fiber even without special bran cereals in the diet.

The Value of Starches

Let's turn from indigestible carbohydrates (fiber) to digestible ones (starches). The main value of starches is to provide energy.

The simple sugars can also provide energy, but somehow starches seem to satisfy the appetite and the bodily demands for energy on a more even basis. In other words, you feel better for a longer time on a fresh vegetable than you do on a candy bar. This may be because the fiber in whole foods causes a steadier increase in blood sugar from the starches in those same foods (which the body converts into sugars).[2] But if you eat simple sugars without fiber accompanying them, you get a faster rise and fall in blood sugar as a response.

Although other nutrients like fat, protein, and alcohol also can be converted into energy, the best source is carbohydrates, particularly the complex starches. We measure the energy of food in terms of calories. The term *calorie* can be a little confusing, but it refers basically to the amount of heat energy released by a portion of food when it's being burned in a special test apparatus. You can think of your body as a kind of metabolic furnace. When it digests and metabolizes food, some of that energy is released as heat. Have you ever noticed on a cold day how you feel much warmer after you've eaten than just before?

In addition to providing body heat, we use energy for activity. This includes visible activities like work, sports, and talking, but it also includes internal activities like breathing and keeping that old heart ticking. At a microscopic level every living cell also uses energy to run its internal machinery, to keep its life processes going.

In chapter 13 we will consider the expenditure of energy through work and exercise. But in this chapter we are focusing on the ingestion of energy from food. You can think of your body as being a savings bank. You cannot take out more money (energy) than you put in; but if you take in more than you use, it gets saved (turns to fat). Although the biochemistry of how this all works is complicated, the important thing to realize is that you need a proper balance of intake to output.

God designed our appetites, our hunger and satiation signal systems, to keep input and output in balance. But as most of us can tell by looking in the mirror or at the average person on the street, appetite control systems fail if we eat the wrong things (concentrated fats and sugars) that our bodies weren't designed to handle and regulate.

Let's say your intake exceeds your output by an average of 100 calories a day. In other words, no more extra food than about one cup of sweetened tea, or a slice of cheese, or a tablespoon of butter, or a medium apple. At that rate you would consume about 3000 extra calories a month. Since a pound of fat equals about 3500 calories, you would thereby gain almost a pound a month, all year long.

It's not that simple, however. At a given meal or in a given day we might eat more than 100 extra calories. But in addition to short-term appetite control, we have long-term bodily awareness of our level of fat. So if we eat way too much at one sitting, we usually eat much less at the next meal or on the next day. For example, if you've been to a banquet or an all-you-can-eat restaurant, you may barely be able to eat anything at the next meal.

Fad diets drastically throw this whole system out of balance. They force you into unbearable hunger and your body thinks it's starving. The minute you go off the diet it's almost impossible to stop eating because the appetite is out of control. You may have struggled for weeks to lose, say, five pounds. But it reappears almost instantly, usually with some extra. After semistarvation, your fat cells are like dried sponges under the water faucet when it first turns on—they soak up those lipids (fats).

I know of a man who went on a fad diet and lost sixty pounds. At first he was elated, but then he gained it all back, plus about five pounds more. A nutritionist wrote me about her own struggle. You'd think a nutritionist, of all people, would know better. But apparently she didn't. Her approach to dieting was simply to cut down on calories but eat the same unbalanced mix of food she had been eating before. She struggled and suffered for two months, and only lost two pounds. When she quit her diet, she gained back four pounds in only one month.

Why do your fat cells reabsorb lipids faster than they lose them? In more primitive societies where food is seasonal, people gorge and fatten up when food is plentiful, but slim down when food is scarce.[3] Because the food supply is not steady, their bodies store up quickly during feast times so they can survive better during famines.

Of course, this principle is of no value in modern societies where food is always plentiful for most people. But our bodily systems don't suddenly change because society has changed. We need to be aware of these mechanisms so that we don't fall into the fad diet trap of sudden starvation followed by rebound fattening up. This rebound principle is one of the key reasons the GIO-KIO plan is so much more helpful than fad diets. This plan allows the body to fill up on the kinds of foods it was designed for. This allows the hunger start-and-stop mechanisms to function properly.

The possibility of rebound is also the reason it's better to improve your diet only a little bit, and then stick to it for the rest of your life, rather than change your diet a lot, but only for a little while. Lasting improvements can give you a permanent benefit, but temporary improvements can leave you worse off than you were before.

Remember: Self-starvation doesn't help! If you are dieting to the extent that you always feel hungry and never satisfied, then you are doing something wrong. You might lose more weight temporarily, but almost certainly you will put that weight back on (plus some bonus pounds). If you fill up on balanced, complex carbohydrates like fresh fruits and vegetables, however, you will be able to keep that weight down and still satisfy your hunger drive.

What the Bible Says

The Bible clearly recognizes the role of food in providing strength and energy. As Psalms 104:14–15 says, God makes "plants for man to cultivate, that he may bring forth food from the earth, and wine to gladden the heart of man, oil to make his face shine, and bread to strengthen man's heart."

Recall again the story of Saul forbidding his troops to stop and eat (1 Samuel 14:24–30). Without a fresh supply of food energy, they soon became so weak that they couldn't sustain the fight properly. They were expending a lot of energy, but consuming no fresh supplies. This doesn't kill you right off the bat, for you have some stored quick energy in the liver and a larger store in body fat and muscle. But if you depend entirely on your own fat for energy, you will feel pretty weak.

There is an important lesson in that episode for us today. Diets too low in carbohydrates and calories can make you feel awful. You may lose weight faster, but much of the loss is muscle rather than fat. *Also, without carbohydrates, you break down the fat incompletely.* This produces a state known as *ketosis,* or an unhealthy overconcentration of ketone bodies (from partial fat breakdown) in the blood.

Ketosis accounts for that weak, groggy, cranky, spacy feeling you get on extreme fad diets. (Ketosis can be very serious for infants and may cause permanent brain damage. With adults, it mostly makes you feel and look sick and miserable.) So you quickly get off the diet and re-form all that fat that you suffered so to break down.

If you follow the GIO-KIO diet correctly, however, you will *not* go into ketosis. You will have plenty of complex carbohydrates to provide you with energy and a feeling of fullness. You will have the carbohydrates you need to break down body fat and burn it *completely*, without producing unwanted ketones.

Think of this steady supply of dietary carbohydrate as incoming oxygen, and your body fat as fuel, say gasoline. Do you know what happens if you run your car in a sealed garage where there isn't enough oxygen to burn the fuel properly? It produces carbon monoxide, a deadly poisonous gas when concentrated. But if you run your car in the presence of plenty of oxygen, there is no problem.

In an analogous way, burning body fat with insufficient carbohydrate intake produces some by-products (ketones) with unpleasant effects (ketosis). But burning it with plenty of complex carbohydrates present allows you to burn up the fat cleanly and completely.

How to Ensure Adequate Energy

The following are the recommended dietary allowances for caloric intake for energy developed by the National Research Council of the National Academy of Sciences. They are average figures only, so your particular needs may vary. In general, the more physically active you are at work and play, the more calories you need.

These figures also assume you want to maintain the body weight you have now. If you want to lose weight, you need to consume less.

Average Daily Calories Required for

Age	Males	Females
1–3	1300	1300
4–6	1700	1700
7–10	2400	2400
11–14	2700	2200
15–18	2800	2100
19–22	2900	2100
23–50	2700	2000
51–74	2400	1800
75+	2050	1600

Note: You do not have to count calories on the GIO-KIO diet. All you need to do is reduce unhealthy food (excess fat, sweets, and protein) and replace it with healthy food (complex carbohydrates). You won't have to keep written records. You won't have to consult all your meals in detailed calorie charts. You won't have to add up numbers and keep track of the totals. *You will not need to eat less than before.* You can eat more and *still lose weight!*

All you have to do is select the right foods, the ones God designed for you, *and* listen to your internal hunger mechanisms, the ones God put there. When you're eating the wrong food or eating in the wrong way, these mechanisms don't work properly. But when you're eating the right food in the right way, these mechanisms will *automatically* get your weight to where it should be.

In other words, when you are hungry, you eat, no matter how many times a day or how much. When you are about full, you stop eating. When you are not hungry, you don't eat at all. It's as simple as that. You will see the excess fat *melt away* as a result.

Since you're not going to count calories, why am I giving you this table of recommended calorie intake?

1. I want you to see how caloric needs rise during growth, but then decline during adulthood. It is crucially important that you understand this decline as metabolism and activity go down. If at thirty you eat as much as you did at twenty, you are going to put on weight. You will add year after year. You will just keep adding fat. Let's say a thirty-year-old woman should eat 2000 calories a day, but she eats instead 2100 as she did when she was twenty. That's only 100 extra calories a day, but 36,500 a year. Since 3500 calories equals one pound of fat, she will put on about ten pounds more fat that year.

2. You should note the gender difference. Men usually need more calories than women. Part of this is the customary difference in activity (this doesn't always hold true, of course). But part depends on basic differences in physique. Because the average male is taller and heavier than the average female (even if they are equally active), the man needs more calories. This difference can cause problems in a family where the wife or mother thinks she should be able to eat as much as the husband or son. She might gain weight on the same diet while he remains the same weight or even loses. (By the way, women who are pregnant should add about 300 additional calories a day, and about 500 more during breast-feeding. At these times, they're eating for two.)

3. I want you to note the magnitude of the number of calories a day you need to maintain weight. If you snack on cheeseburgers (525 calories), milk shakes (335 calories), and cheesecake (280 calories per slice), you can quickly meet or even exceed these recommended daily totals. But if you snack on grapes (4 calories each, or about 80 for a bunch), apples (80 calories), or celery (5 calories per stalk), you can eat your fill and still come in way below the total to maintain weight. In other words, *you can enjoy all you want of the right foods and still lose weight!*

Don't be like Max, who is married, forty-two, and a registered nurse practitioner. He says, "I want to weigh only one hundred eighty pounds so my clothes will fit better. I think I would look better, too." But he's going about this the wrong way. He gives up all his favorite foods and reports, "I stay on a diet almost continuously." The main result, however, is that he feels frequently hungry, frequently irritable, and loses patience with others. That's no way to live!

Don't waste time counting calories. Select the right foods, eat only when you're hungry, and then don't worry about anything else. Just praise God and eat your fill. You'll get your weight in order, cut out that bulging fat, *and* feel and look better. The best part of all is that eating the right foods not only gets you slim and keeps you slim, but keeps you vigorous, healthy, and more alive. It helps make *you* become the special person you really are inside.

Let the butterfly out of the cocoon *now!*

COMPLEX CARBOHYDRATES *ENERGIZE YOU*

11

The Need for Water

Water. Most of the earth's surface is covered with it. The atmosphere we breathe is usually filled with it. We begin life as developing embryos floating in it. And the majority of our body weight consists of plain, ordinary water. Water composes about 60 percent of a young man's total body weight and about 50 percent of a young woman's,[1] though these proportions decline slightly with age.[2] This means that a 120-pound woman may be carrying about 60 pounds of water, while a 150-pound man may be holding 90 pounds.

Why don't we slosh around like water jugs when we walk? The reason is that only a minor portion of all this water exists in an obviously fluid, pourable state like blood. There is not only water outside of and between the body's living cells, but within them as well. The blood supply accounts for only perhaps three quarts of water in the average person, while about nine and one-half quarts exist in the tiny spaces between cells, and an amazing twenty-five quarts rest within the individual cells.[3]

If the normal human body contains more water than anything else, this precious fluid obviously must be important.

Bodily Uses of Water

Each living cell requires water within it to survive. Water composes part of the structure of each cell and allows the cell to carry out its various vital life functions.

Most nutrients can dissolve in water, thus enabling the blood to carry them. Then the water stuck between cells can convey nutrients from the blood to the cells, and waste products from the cells back to the blood again. Also, the water within cells can carry nutrients and transport waste products to the cell membranes for ejection. In other words, this vast bodily waterway serves a variety of transport functions.

Water plays a role in chemical reactions, including those related to digestion. It takes water, for instance, to help split ingested proteins into their component building blocks. Conversely, when the body forms new proteins from these blocks, as in the formation of muscle, water is released. Without water, these essential reactions couldn't occur.

Water provides the bulk of perspiration, which is essential for control of body temperature. We do not perspire only because of nervous tension, as some deodorant ads imply. We perspire to release body heat and keep our temperatures from rising abnormally. The sweat glands release water onto the surface of the skin, and as it evaporates, it takes heat away from the body. One quart, or about two pounds, of water evaporating as sweat can carry away 544 calories of body heat.[4] Thus the greater the body's heat, due both to external heat (room or outdoor temperature) and internal heat production (as from exercise), the more the need for perspiration. In heavy exercise a person can lose two to four quarts (four to eight pounds) of water as sweat *in one hour*.[5] Even without exercise, people sweat continuously throughout the day to lose body heat.

Finally, water serves as a lubricant within the body. For instance, the average person secretes one to two quarts of saliva a day.[6] The enzymes in saliva help to digest food. The water helps to moisten food and lets it slide into the digestive tract easier. By the way, the huge volume of water secreted as saliva is not all lost to the body but is reabsorbed in the intestines. Water also serves a lubricating role in the joints, where it helps to cushion them during body movements.[7]

The Hazards of Dehydration

Dehydration refers to a loss of water or partial drying of the body. In light of the many bodily needs for water, it should not be surprising that dehydration can be harmful. Most people don't realize that even when plentiful fluids are available for drinking, they still can get dehydrated. People assume their thirst drive will get them to drink whenever they should and as much as they should. Unfortunately, this is not always true. If the hunger drive often fails to keep body weight at the normal level, it really shouldn't come as a surprise that the thirst drive often fails to keep the right amount of water in the body.

This usually occurs when exercising, especially in warm weather. People who are exercising may think they are drinking enough, but they probably sweat even more than they take in. In a fairly short time they can lose about a pound or two of water (one to two pints).

The symptoms caused by dehydration depend on the amount of water lost:

1. Losing 1 to 5 percent of body weight in water (1 to 6 pounds for a 120-pound person) could produce these effects:[8] flushed skin, loss of appetite, general discomfort, and behavioral decrements.
2. Losing 6 to 10 percent of body weight in water (7 to 12 pounds for a 120-pound person), could cause these more serious symptoms:[9] headache, dizziness, difficulty speaking, and difficulty walking. Remember, it would be possible to lose this much water in even one hour of heavy exercise in a hot environment if one didn't drink some replacement fluids.
3. Losing 11 to 20 percent of body weight in water (13 to 24 pounds for a 120-pound person) could cause these conditions:[10] shriveled skin, loss of urination, mental delirium, and loss of muscle control.

Exceeding a 20 percent loss could cause death. This level of dehydration is unlikely to occur except in unusual circumstances, as when someone is lost in the desert, or perhaps when an elderly person remains at home alone without air conditioning in the summer.

Such extreme levels of dehydration are rare in modern society, but probably everyone has experienced signs of mild dehydration, possibly quite often, without realizing the cause. Recent studies show that mild dehydration of just 2 or 3 percent body weight loss in water can affect mental performance.[11,12] The person may feel vaguely uncomfortable, unmotivated, and "out of it" mentally without even realizing why. His heart rate may go up considerably and he may lose his ability to tolerate heat.[13]

There are some long-term risks to dehydration as well. One study, for instance, found that even one experience of severe dehydration early in life led to a fourfold increase in cataract blindness later.[14] Having two experiences of severe dehydration led to a twenty-onefold increase in such eye problems later. The potential of dehydration to cause serious harm to one's health is not immediately obvious but is very real.

Achieving Water Balance

Theoretically it sounds simple to match water intake with water loss. The problem is that there are methods both for intake and loss of which we often aren't aware. And as already noted, the thirst drive does not perfectly control water balance, particularly when heavy perspiration causes a rapid loss of body water.

Ways Body Water Is Lost

1. *Perspiration.* Everyone sweats. When in hot environments and exercising, the loss may be dramatic, up to several pounds of water an hour.
2. *Breathing.* Water vapor is expelled with every breath, a process clearly seen in cold weather when the breath immediately clouds up in a miniature "fog." The total

lost this way may be less than one pint per day under resting conditions. But it may be as much as two to three ounces per hour with strenuous exercise when one is breathing heavier.

3. *Body waste.* Some water is lost with the feces, and quite a bit with urine. With diarrhea the capacity of the intestines to reabsorb water is temporarily lost, and the person can lose a considerable amount in a short time. This is one of the more common causes of dehydration among infants and small children. Also various diseases and diuretic (urine-promoting) drugs can cause water loss in the urine to be greater than usual.

4. *Chemical reactions.* Some water is lost, or at least tied up temporarily, through various chemical reactions. In digesting proteins, for instance, some water molecules leave the liquid state and become part of the amino acids, the building blocks of protein.

Ways Body Water Is Gained

1. *Drinking fluids.* I was raised to drink plain water when thirsty, and it always amazes me to find people who never touch the stuff. Some people get all their fluids from juice, milk, soda, and other flavored beverages. While this approach can take care of one's fluid needs, since all beverages consist mostly of water, it costs more and can add significantly to caloric intake (unless only diet drinks are consumed). An eight-ounce glass of whole milk, for instance, provides 150 calories, while eight ounces of orange juice adds 110 calories.

Milk and juice certainly are nutritious, and some of each is quite valuable. But if one consistently quenches thirst only with such beverages, hundreds of unnecessary calories will be added to his daily intake. One of the most interesting talks I heard at the North American Association for the Study of Obesity's 1987 conference in Boston dealt with this topic. Dr. David Booth of the University of Birmingham, England, maintains that routine use of high-calorie beverages is one of the most common and least recognized causes of obesity. People realize that solid foods contain calories, but they often act as if beverages didn't. But this just isn't so.

Pure drinking water, on the other hand, is absolutely calorie free. Water may also contain small amounts of nutritious minerals like calcium and magnesium, not to mention that cavity preventer, fluoride. As a minimum, each person should drink two to three quarts of fluid daily, and ideally only a small portion of this should come in the form of flavored drinks that contain calories.

2. *Eating food.* Some foods like fruits are juicy and obviously contain lots of water. But even apparently "dry" foods like beans, nuts, and bread contain significant amounts of water. Cooked beans, for instance, contain around 65 percent water, while whole-wheat bread contains 38 percent water, and even "dry" Swiss cheese contains 42 percent. All told, food intake may provide up to half of one's daily water ingestion.

3. *Chemical reactions.* Just as some biochemical activities require water, some release water back into the system. For instance, the production of both fat and protein in the body releases water.

Factors Increasing the Need for Water

1. *Exercise.* The more exercise, the greater the heat production in the body, and the greater the loss of water in perspiration. If the exerciser doesn't get this extra water, his or her ability to perform will decline.

2. *External heat.* The greater the external temperature, the more the need for water as perspiration. For every 5°F increase in temperature over 85°F, an adult should consume about one pint of fluid more per day, even if not exercising.[15]

3. *Dry climate.* The drier the outside air, the quicker water evaporates from the surface of the skin.

4. *High altitude.* The greater one's elevation above the

earth's surface, the less the air pressure, and the easier it is to get dehydrated. Jet passengers, for instance, should take care to drink more than usual so they'll feel better and more alert when they land.

5. *Illness.* Certain illnesses increase the need for body water. For instance, a fever of 4°F above normal (a temperature of about 103°F) increases the need for water intake by about one pint per day.[16] Illnesses like diarrhea that cause a fluid loss increase the need for water intake.

6. *Injuries.* Cuts and wounds involving bleeding or oozing and burns all increase the need for fluid intake.

7. *Diet.* Certain compounds like alcohol and caffeine tend to increase urine production and the need for replacement water.

Water Excess

Some people retain too much body fluid, resulting in edema (swelling) and bloating. Such a condition may be caused by a serious heart or kidney condition or something similar that requires the immediate attention of a physician.

Having drastically too much body water can even result in a condition known as *water intoxication.*[17] This may cause weakness, convulsions, and even coma. Such a condition is caused by disease, however, and a normal person could not reach this point simply by drinking too much, for his kidneys would excrete all the extra rather quickly.

On the other hand, deliberate overdrinking could temporarily throw off the acid-base balance of the blood and cause an altered mental state that some consider to be a type of "high." I have heard of institutionalized drug addicts who, deprived of their usual kicks, frantically overdrink in the attempt to reach this state, which lasts only as long as they can drink more than their kidneys put out.

Although no normal person needs to worry about drinking too much water, it's likely too little water will be consumed under certain circumstances unless one takes care to drink enough fluid.

WATER IS
THE MOST
IMPORTANT
NUTRIENT OF ALL

12

Breaking the Tyranny of Gluttony

This is the tough one, isn't it? In recent chapters we looked at reducing excess fat, sugar, and protein. It's not too hard to cut down on one of those as long as you increase one or more of the others. Some fad diets go that route: They'll rule out sweets, but increase protein to dangerous levels.

That's no good. As we saw in chapter 5, the key to healthy eating is more balance in your diet, not less. But now we're looking at controlling your total caloric intake regardless of how balanced your diet is. That's scary.

But as I've said before, you are *not* going to be forcing yourself into unbearable hunger on this diet. You are *not* going to just give up foods you like. You will need to cut down on some. But even then, you will practice *replacement* rather than simple deprivation.

We are not talking about eating less than you need so that you suffer. We are talking about *not eating more than you need*, so you will stop gaining weight year after year. If you stick to this diet and health plan, if your weight is now reasonable, you can *stop* the creeping weight gain that most adults experience. Even if you choose not to lose a pound on this diet, but just manage to prevent future weight gain, I believe you are a success. In other words, a diet that makes you healthy and prevents weight gain for the rest of your life is great, even if you don't lose umpteen pounds and look like Twiggy now.

Fad diets can't help you cope with this problem of hunger. If your weight goes down due to self-starvation, it bounces right back up again like a rubber ball. These diets in the long run make more, not fewer, people into gluttons. It's always feast or famine. After a certain period of unbearable famine the person feasts back on more pounds than he starved off.

Susan wrote me about her sister. It seems the sister "normally eats large quantities like a man." In other words, she usually overeats. But then she gets scared about her creeping obesity and plunges into a fad diet every couple of months. As she gets sick of the diet, she goes right back to her old habits. The result is that "she never loses weight."

Susan herself, on the other hand, follows the GIO-KIO concept of cutting down on fats, sweets, and protein. But she doesn't go hungry. Instead, she replaces the lost foods with plenty of fresh vegetables and fruits at lunch and dinner. The result? In less than two months, she has lost nine pounds, declining from 136 to 127, which is about right for her.

Susan says that the hardest part was giving up ice cream, which she loves dearly. My reply is don't give up all of your favorite foods. Don't force yourself into a position where you hate and resent your diet, because you'll soon quit. Instead of giving up your treasured foods, just cut down serving sizes or frequency. Replace the missing portions of treats with fresh, tasty foods that are better for your health.

With this approach, you can lose your excess weight even when conditions all around you don't seem right. Bill, who is single and twenty-three years old, follows the plan of cutting down on red meat and junk food snacks and replaces these with fresh fruits and vegetables. This way he lost ten pounds, even though his schedule often forced him to eat out, where it's harder to control what you consume. His best friend did even better. The friend is a single parent with a four-year-old daughter and lots of stress. Yet, when he got with the program, he lost twenty pounds! These true stories illustrate that we can break free of the tyranny of gluttony.

Avoid Overeating

One edition of *Webster's* Dictionary defines a *glutton* as "one who indulges to excess in eating." Why do we indulge in excess? There are many possible reasons:

1. *Habit.* In the teenage years we can usually eat like pigs and not gain much body fat. Metabolism, activity, and energy use are high then. For a while we are still growing. But when all of these processes slow down, starting in young adulthood and continuing until the end of life, we may still eat like teenagers. We don't really plan to overeat, but we do. Our bodies have played a dirty trick on us, and we haven't realized how to stop it. Once formed, habits are hard to break. (If you fit into this category, don't worry. Later we'll see a great way to help reverse this process of declining metabolism.)

2. *Social pressure.* Many families worry if their babies don't eat "enough." Throughout all the years of growing up, these parents keep pushing food at kids, thinking and complaining that something is wrong if they don't eat it all. I'll never forget what happened to my wife and me when we initially took our firstborn son to church. Another set of parents was there with their newborn boy, too. We looked at each other. Our son was slender, but muscular and bright. He ate well, and we were always careful to give him a balanced diet both before birth (via my wife's diet) and afterward. We looked at the other boy and thought he was drastically obese, a real butterball who must be overfed day and night. This other couple, though, had different ideas. They looked at our boy in alarm, saying, "Don't you ever feed that kid? He looks like he's starving to death!"

Likewise, often hosts and hostesses at social functions act offended if guests don't eat a certain amount. Friends may encourage you to join them in treats, eating out, or snacking. Once you begin a diet and start to change your eating habits, you can count on having some people notice the difference and not like it. Somehow the fact that you now get just a single-scoop dish of ice cream rather than a triple-scoop cone as usual (and as they still do) seems to offend or threaten them. It's as if you are challenging them to cut down, too, and they don't like it!

Learn to overcome this kind of opposition with a joke and a laugh. Don't make an issue out of it, or it will make sticking to your diet and health plan more difficult. Above all, don't preach at your friends about the evils or risks of gluttony or you might lose some friends! If you are to have a positive effect on your friends' health, it will not be because you collar them and nag them to join you. It will come about by their seeing your example and wanting to know more about how you got so slim, healthy, alert, and active all of a sudden. Then you can tell them about the GIO-KIO plan or give them a copy of this book.

Remember: Don't eat when you're not hungry. This also applies to that familial adage, "Clean your plate." It's better to save or even throw out the last few forkfuls of something than to ingest more calories than your body needs. Some people eat every last crumb because they "hate to waste food." Naturally, we should all avoid willful waste of food. Ideally, we should prepare and serve only as much as we need. But if there's a little left on the plate and you force yourself to eat it when you don't need it, that's wasting food, too, but in a different way.

3. Stress. We all experience stress, more at some times than at others. Although stress affects the whole body, in particular it drains certain neurochemicals from the brain.[1] In time this causes an uncomfortable feeling

that I refer to as being "zonked." We feel wasted and worn out, unwilling to continue the struggle. But eating carbohydrate-rich snacks and sweets seems to calm us down and make us feel better.[2] There's nothing wrong with eating *a little more when under stress*, because that's when your body needs a little more. But if you use major quantities of food to calm down, you're using food like a tranquilizer, a drug.[3]

4. *Compensation.* Sometimes we feel deprived in life. The divorced parent feels the loss of love and support. The man passed over for a promotion feels frustrated and cheated. The student who gets a lesser grade than she deserves or doesn't make the track team feels slighted or left out. At such times, we often feel a temptation to overindulge in food as a way of "paying ourselves back" for the misfortune we're suffering. But again, this is using food more like a drug than a gift of God.

5. *Pleasure.* Sometimes we eat more than we should simply because it tastes good. It feels good. We like that second slice of lemon meringue pie or second chocolate milk shake. There's nothing wrong with enjoying food up to a point. It is, after all, a gift of God. But when we overindulge we forget one simple fact: The extra strawberry shortcake makes us feel good for a few moments, as we're eating it. But it causes far more pain for a far longer time afterward. It adds to our weight problem; it isn't healthy. We feel sluggish and robbed of the energy we need to lead happy, active lives of service to God and to His people. Next time you're faced with the temptation of a huge banana split or butterscotch sundae, ask yourself which is more important, a few moments of oral pleasure or the lasting rewards of being healthy and trim.

Now that we know *why* we indulge in excess, just what is excess, anyway? There's nothing wrong with limited quantities of the dessert foods I just mentioned. I like them as much as you. Those are not foods to look down on as being somehow inferior, *as long as they are consumed in reasonable amounts.* The problem comes from excess use, of which these are some signs:

1. We eat even when we don't feel hungry, just to fulfill some other psychological or social need.
2. We let the dessert or junk food displace more healthy foods from our diets. We might have so many between-meal snacks of the sweet and fat variety that we don't have much appetite for balanced meals of more healthy food.
3. We don't want others to know how much we're eating. We eat in secret or try to conceal how much is missing from the family larder.
4. We rely on food like a drug, to make us feel better.
5. When upset, rather than when hungry, we reach for a snack.
6. We eat until we feel unpleasantly full or bloated.
7. We eat so much that our weight keeps climbing, year after year.
8. We eat because someone else wants us to, even if we don't feel like it.
9. We eat just "to finish it" or clean the plate, even though we know we're already full.
10. We eat so much that we feel guilty rather than grateful to God.
11. We eat so much that we want to make ourselves throw up rather than digest the food (i.e., bulimia).

Most people probably already know whether or not they are overeating. It's not so much the knowledge of gluttony they need, but the knowledge of how to break free.

What the Bible Says

The Bible does not speak kindly of gluttony. Proverbs 23:2 says to put a knife to your throat if you are given to appetite [gluttony]. In other words, gluttony as good as kills you.

Proverbs 23:20–21 says, "Be not among winebibbers, or among gluttonous eaters of meat; for the drunkard and the glutton will come to poverty, and drowsiness will clothe a man with rags." This passage says some scary things. It likens gluttons to alcoholics. In both cases, the person feels a compulsion to consume; he has lost control. The Bible says there are serious consequences to either form of dependence. There is an economic cost, because food and wine have a price, and there is a cost on behavior, mood, and personality. As research done in the last few years shows, eating too much can make you drowsy, that is, weak or groggy.[4] The Bible recognized that thousands of years ago!

Philippians 3:19 talks about people who dwell too much on food: ". . . their god is the belly, and they glory in their shame, with minds set on earthly things." This to me sounds like serious gluttons, epicures, or maybe bulimics. They revel in filling their stomachs, but in a perverse, shameful way. This misuse of one of God's gifts stands in the way of spiritual growth and development.

Jesus put the problem in a nutshell when He said, "Truly, truly, I say to you, every one who commits sin is a slave to sin" (John 8:34). Bulimics and others with food compulsions certainly know the truth of that one! The habit holds them tightly in its grip; even knowing and suffering the consequences of their excess does not enable them to break free. The situation seems almost, but not quite, hopeless.

There is the Gospel! God can cleanse us from all sin. He can free us from the power of it. He can take the noose right off our necks. As Matthew 6:25 says, we shouldn't worry about (that is, be slaves to) food. We should trust God and allow Him to provide.

One way is to listen to our own bodies. We can become attuned to the hunger mechanisms that God built in. When we really are physically hungry, we should eat. We shouldn't deprive ourselves indefinitely according to the schedule of some fad diet. When we are *not* hungry, we shouldn't eat. God built those hunger and satiation mechanisms to keep our body weights normal, not too high or too low.

Okay, but in our society sometimes we have to go out to lunch or sit down to dinner according to a schedule, whether hungry or not. Put in your appearance, but don't eat any more than you need. Be polite, but don't eat to excess. It's just not worth it.

Seek Help From God

If you are plagued by habitual overeating and are having trouble cutting down, ask God for help. Shifting from poor eating habits to good ones takes time. For a while you may feel unsure of yourself. Sometimes you will stumble and fall back into the old patterns. But "after you have suffered a little while, the God of all grace, who has called you to his eternal glory in Christ, will himself restore, establish, and strengthen you" (1 Peter 5:10). If you come to God in faith, with trust, you *will* win a victory over food habits and compulsions. Pray about this problem, if you have it, every day.

I know a lay preacher and Sunday-school teacher named Robert who takes this seriously. And prayer has made all the difference in the world to him. A few years ago, he weighed 213 pounds. He was told he had to lose twenty pounds or lose his job. This made him take his diet seriously. Soon he began to lose a little weight. His pants started to get looser and people praised and encouraged him. So he kept going, not just to lose the minimum to get by, but to lose all he needed to look completely slim, muscular, and healthy. In just six months, he lost forty-four pounds! Now, at age thirty-eight, he looks like a trim athlete. His wife got motivated, in part by seeing his success. She lost 130 pounds in less than a year! Now in her mid-thirties, she could pass for a model.

Other Techniques for Appetite Control

In addition to prayer and Bible study, the following are psychological techniques to help you control your appetite:

1. *Don't wait a long time between eating.* Many people try to hold out until they're too ravenous to wait any longer. That's *not* a good idea. It tends to make you eat too fast and too much when you finally do start to chow down. Instead, eat many small meals or frequent snacks (the nondessert kind) throughout the day as soon as you become aware of mounting hunger. Your snack may only need to be as large as half an apple or a stick of celery. It may have almost no calories. But it will help you keep your appetite down to manageable levels.

2. *Eat slowly.* When you gobble down food, particularly high-fat food, you can eat far too much before your hunger stop mechanism catches up with you. This is a complicated scientific matter, but the essence is as follows: It takes time for your stomach and intestines to respond to food you've eaten. There are receptors in the stomach that respond to it stretching as it fills up; there are receptors that respond to digestive hormones and other chemicals being called into play; and there are receptors that indicate the absorption of digested nutrients into the system. All this takes time. If you wolf down your food, you will go past the point of satiation (being full) *before* your body can catch up with you and tell you that. In other words, your brain doesn't realize that you've already eaten enough. It tells you you're still hungry, and so you keep eating.

   But if you eat slowly enough, your body can keep better track of how much you've eaten and when you're satiated. Also, eating more slowly allows you to enjoy eating more. Furthermore, chewing more thoroughly greatly aids the digestive process. I believe most people chew too little and eat too fast, and thus cause themselves needless indigestion and gastrointestinal distress.

3. *Start the meal by drinking lots of water and eating lower calorie foods like plain bread and salad.* This gives you a chance to fill up on a more balanced diet

before you get to the banana pudding or ice cream sundae. If you start with high-calorie items like fatty meats, you will tend to consume too many calories, and yet you will feel no fuller than if you did it the other way.

4. *Stop eating a given meal or snack a little before you feel completely full.* In the next few minutes your digestive system and brain will catch up to you and tell you that you are full. On the other hand, if you keep eating until you definitely feel full, over the next half hour you will feel overly satiated as your brain catches up with the overload you packed in. This can make you feel uncomfortable and groggy for hours after eating.

5. *Always leave at least a little something on your plate as a symbol that you can say "no" to food.* If you are like I am, you were raised to feel proud for cleaning your plate, whether you were hungry for the food or not. That approach encourages overeating. Don't waste food, but leave a bite or so to prove that you can be firm. For the same reason, it's better to start with a small first helping of something and then go back for more, rather than starting with a mountain of food that you feel obligated to chow down.

6. *Exercise.* This is the best way to help control appetite (more on this in chapter 13).

7. *Have others encourage you.* Let your good friends and trusted family members know you are on the GIO-KIO diet. Ask them to pray for you, to reward you for showing restraint at the table, for replacing junk foods with healthful foods, for looking slimmer and healthier as your body thrives on this fitness plan.

Martha, for instance, who is a thirty-three-year-old secretary, tried various diets before. But as she said, she had "no willpower—I could never stay on one for more than a week." But then she asked for, and got, the help of her family. She had them fighting the fight with her, rooting for her to win. They also avoided serving tempting foods that could be her downfall. The result? She lost twenty-three pounds in just eight weeks. And she has kept it off for two years, without gaining a single pound back! One of her neighbors did even better, she says, but it took him longer. In a year he took off thirty pounds!

8. *Prayer.* If other humans can help you, imagine how much more God can! I've mentioned this before, but it's worth repeating again and again. Terry is thirty-seven, married, and the father of two. He has a vibrant personality and works actively in his church, especially as an avid supporter of the choir. He is five feet, six inches tall and used to weigh 239 pounds. He says, "My dietary habits directly affect my weight, health, and mental attitude. It is a spiritual struggle that I need to ask God's help for *daily*." I asked him what were his main reasons for wanting to lose weight, and he said, "It looked disgusting. It was a disadvantage for my back problems. It was not a proper way to care for the body God gave me." Terry had a good attitude toward making some long overdue dietary changes. When he did, he learned to substitute healthy foods for junk foods, to avoid binges, and to avoid eating out of emotional stress or boredom rather than hunger. The key to his approach, however, was this: "Prayer is of the utmost importance!" And the result? It took him a year, but he lost *over 100 pounds!* Now he has not an extra ounce of fat visible on his trim frame.

Is this the kind of change in your life that you need?

DON'T EAT
MORE
THAN YOU NEED
BUT DO
EAT ENOUGH

Section III

Burning Up Calories

13

The Fun Way to Lose Weight

Most fad diets stress deprivation—horrible, painful deprivation. They leave out the most important weight-loss secret of all: exercise.

I know, I know, memories of dreaded gym classes make that a scary word. Sometimes you can hardly face walking across the room, much less running a marathon. You know how stupid some of those joggers look out there. And there's no way you're going to make yourself into a candidate for the orthopedic ward.

Good. You're absolutely right. I agree with you. There's no point even thinking about starting a strenuous, unpleasant athletic program that you hate. If you're looking at it that way, you'll soon quit. And you might hurt yourself in the meantime.

Forget all about the regimented gym class, forget all about huffing and puffing until your knees wobble, your bones ache, and you think your heart will explode. Instead, think fun.

One man's fun exercise is another man's torment. Don't think about what's fun for me or your neighbor or your children if it's something you dislike. What do you like? What activity do you think is fun enough that you're willing to do it at least three times a week for at least twenty or thirty minutes at a time?

There's got to be something. If you are now out of shape, of
course, you should consult your physician before starting any
kind of new exercise program. If you don't have in mind a
satisfactory kind of exercise, discuss some options with him or
her. The following chart lists different kinds of activities. But it
also tells you the approximate number of calories per minute
that you can burn with each activity.

Calories Spent Per Minute for Various Activities

Resting, Standing, and Walking

Resting in bed	1.2	Kneeling	1.4
Sitting	1.4	Squatting	2.2
Sitting, reading	1.4	Walking, indoors	3.4
Sitting, eating	1.6	Walking, outdoors	6.1
Sitting, playing cards	1.7	Walking, downstairs	7.6
Standing	1.6	Walking, upstairs	20.0
Standing, light activity	2.8	Standing, showering	3.7

Working Around the Home

Washing clothes	2.9	Mopping floors	5.3
Hanging laundry	4.7	Sweeping floors	1.7
Bringing in laundry	3.2	Scrubbing floors	6.0
Machine sewing	1.5	Shaking carpets	6.4
Ironing clothes	4.2	Peeling vegetables	2.9
Making beds	5.3	Stirring, mixing foods	3.0

Do It Yourself

Sawing wood	6.9	Pushing wheelbarrow	5.2
Planing wood	8.6	Chopping wood	4.9
Carrying tools	3.6	Stacking wood	6.1
Shoveling	7.1	Drilling	7.0

Sports and Hobbies

Football	10.1	Badminton	2.8
Basketball	8.6	Rowing	8.0
Ping-Pong	4.8	Sailing	2.6
Swimming	12.1	Playing pool	3.0

Golfing	5.5	Dancing	4.0
Tennis	7.0	Horseback riding	3.0
Bowling	8.1	Cycling	8.0

Source: Are You Really Serious About Losing Weight? 8th ed. (Philadelphia: Pennwalt, 1975), p. 21.

This list groups activities by type. It also gives you an idea of how strenuous various activities are, compared with each other. The more calories per minute an activity requires, the more strenuous it is.

Many things on this list don't count as exercise, of course. Things like resting in bed and sitting are included for comparison with football and swimming. As you can see, even resting burns calories, because our bodies are metabolic furnaces that keep burning up energy to maintain the activities that sustain life. Just keeping our hearts pumping and our lungs expanding requires work and energy. All activities of living burn some calories; not all count as exercise.

While you're still sitting quietly and reading, take your pulse right now. Count the number of beats in sixty seconds. If you're healthy and have been sitting still for at least several minutes, your pulse should be somewhere around sixty to eighty, depending on age and sex and individual differences.

To get any real benefit of exercise to your cardiovascular system (heart and blood vessels), you've got to get that heart rate significantly higher for a while. *Not too high,* of course. I don't want you to start going wild and kill yourself (literally) by doing too much too soon. Even if you don't die, you can suffer some painful injuries that way. Such injuries from ill-planned exercise can prevent you from doing even your ordinary activities for a while, and that would make your weight problem even worse.

How high should your pulse rate get during major exercise? Consult the following table.

Exercise Pulse Rates

Age	Target Zone
20	120–150
25	117–146
30	114–142
35	111–138
40	108–135
45	105–131
50	102–127
55	99–123
60	96–120
65	93–116
70	90–113

"Target Zone" is the pulse or heart rate in beats per minute. Exercise that sustains that target zone level for 30 minutes should be undertaken at least three times a week. Persons over 40 who have not been exercising regularly should consult a doctor before embarking on such a program.

Source: "The Fight Against Heart Disease," *FDA Consumer* (February, 1986), Department of Health and Human Services Publication No. (FDA) 86-1126, p. 5.

These are average, suggested figures. During an exercise session you don't have to stay strictly within those guidelines. Don't keep monitoring yourself, for that would be boring and would interfere with your enjoyment of the activity itself.

On the other hand, it would be good to check your pulse rate about once per exercise session. Pick a time around the maximum intensity of activity. If the activity is like jogging or walking, you don't even have to quit to do this. Just find your pulse (at the wrist or neck) and count for six seconds. Then multiply by ten (to get the normal count per minute). You will only get a rough estimate counting for six seconds, but that should be enough for our purposes.

For activities like tennis, where you can't stop in the middle even for a second to take your pulse, wait until the moment when you finish the activity. But take your pulse immediately then, because the healthy heart begins to slow down rapidly as soon as you stop exercising.

Don't worry if your peak pulse rate is a little higher than these figures, as long as you don't continuously stay above them during exercise. I often jog for my exercise and in the early phases of a run, my pulse rate fits nicely into my target zone. But I live on a hill, and I like to finish my run heading up that hill. That makes my pulse go up much faster. I get well above my target zone, but for a short time (less than a minute). When I feel that it's getting too high, I stop running and walk. I go by how I feel, not by how far I made it up the hill. In other words, I don't aim for some arbitrary goal like running to the top no matter how much it hurts. I'm not trying to win the Boston Marathon. I'm just out there trying to have a little fun; I'm trying to keep in shape and stay healthy.

If you are now out of shape, I recommend you do *not* exceed the target zone at all for several weeks at least. Start low on any exercise program and work your way up gradually. In my case, I jogged regularly for about a year before even trying to run up hills like the one where I live now.

Remember, you're not trying to break any records. You're not trying to push yourself to the limit. You're not trying to see how fast you can improve.

Pick activities that you can enjoy sticking to for the rest of your life. And since you've got that much time to enjoy the activity, go at the speed and for the time that feels good to you now. Don't ever let anybody else tell you that you should go faster or push yourself harder than what feels good to you. You're doing it to have fun and stay healthy, *not* to please anyone else or meet someone else's standards.

The Glorious Benefits of Exercise

I already told you how as a young man I quickly put on forty pounds of fat. One reason was my lack of exercise. I wasn't completely sedentary, and I did work hard. But I quickly got out of the exercise habit that had been drilled into me in high school and college physical education classes.

There came a time when I don't believe I could have walked a mile comfortably (now I can run four or five easily). I remember when I taught as a college professor, one of my students said I should get more exercise. I told her I was too busy to do that, and I meant it. I didn't think I had time to go outside and run or play golf or chop wood.

What I learned later is that exercise pays off huge dividends in making you feel better and letting you work more efficiently. It actually *saves* time! You get more real work done in the eight or twelve hours you have left than you would in the eight and one-half or twelve and one-half hours you would have by skipping exercise.

I took several months to work up to this point, but now I exercise every morning and every evening for about half an hour per session. Sometimes I even go out a third time in the middle of the day. I may jog, I may go for a brisk walk, or I may go for a leisurely family walk. At least three times a week I do calisthenics indoors. My neighbors think I'm crazy, because I go out in the snow, in the rain, or in the dark. When I spent a week crossing the Atlantic Ocean in a cramped submarine studying navy food problems, I found a small corner of space and jogged in place.

Am I a lunatic or a fanatic? No, it just feels so good that I don't want to stop. If someone made me stay idle and indoors all day, I would feel wretched and apathetic. You see, exercise has lots going for it and *nothing* going against it, as long as you're careful and don't overdo it or hurt yourself. My personal pattern, of course, may sound like too much or like the wrong thing for you. You decide what you like and do it. It doesn't matter what it is as long as it gets your pulse rate up around those target figures for at least twenty to thirty minutes at least three times a week.

Here are a few of the benefits you can expect from that degree (or more) of exercise:

1. *Exercise burns calories.* You've already seen the chart that shows the calories per minute you burn with various exercises. Let's look at it now in a different way. Eating and drinking brings in calories. Exercise can burn them off *before they turn to fat.* That's the best way to kill those calories, rather than after they've changed your shape. Here's a chart that shows how much exercise it takes to "pay for" or use up the calories of various foods:

Minutes Per Activity

Food	Calories	Bowl-ing	Walk-ing	Tennis	Bicycl-ing	Stair Climbing	Run-ning
Large apple	100	23	19	14	12	10	5
Orange juice	120	27	23	17	15	12	6
Cereal/milk and sugar	200	45	38	28	24	20	10
Tuna sandwich	278	63	53	39	34	28	18
Hamburger	350	80	67	49	43	36	18
Spaghetti	396	90	76	56	48	40	20

Source: David R. Swarner, ed., *Planning Meals to Lose Weight* (Bristol, Tennessee: Beecham Laboratories), p. 7.

The first column provides the average number of calories in a typical serving of the given food. The remaining columns tell you how many minutes of each exercise it takes to burn off those calories. For instance, twelve minutes of bicycling will use up the 100 calories you get from eating a large apple. Eighteen minutes of running will use up the 350 calories you eat in a hamburger, and so on.

This approach of using exercise to burn calories
works. Michael, for example, was unwilling to make any
dietary changes. He did not follow the complete plan
outlined here. The main thing he did was engage in
regular exercise. He lost eight pounds in just a few days.
And he has kept every ounce of it off since then. He says,
"Exercise is the most important secret of dieting
success."

Not only does exercise burn calories, it forces your
body to burn the right ones. If you simply diet but do not
exercise, your body will consume its own muscle in
addition to fat. But if you exercise as well, you will avoid
most of the usual muscle loss due to dieting, but increase
the loss of fat.

2. *Exercise suppresses the appetite.* If you're having any
trouble with your appetite, you have another reason to
hit the tennis court, jogging trail, or exercise bike. If
you've got cravings for chocolate, ice cream, or whatever, a brisk walk will help cure you. It's paradoxical,
because you would think that spending more calories
would make you hungrier. But it doesn't. This is all
part of the innate hunger/satiation system that God
built into our bodies to regulate our weight at normal,
healthy levels. It's when we quit exercising that appetite grows by leaps and bounds, that we lose control
over the system, and that fat appears. Use exercise to
get back in control of your physical condition.

Dr. M. K., for instance, wrote me that he tried a fad
diet plan which involved no exercise. He lost eight
pounds with great effort, but then added it all back in
just two months. Even with a diet plan inferior to the
GIO-KIO plan, he could have kept most or all of that
weight off simply by adding exercise.

3. *Exercise increases the metabolic rate.* Exercise gives
one blessing after another. Not only do you burn more
calories while you exercise, you burn more even afterward. In other words, if you're just sitting after a good
handball game, you're still burning more calories per

minute than if you had been sitting all day. Even that
night, while asleep, you will burn more calories than if
you had skipped exercise all day. It sounds miraculous,
too good to be true. But it *is* true. Exercise gives you a
more finely tuned machine that burns fuel more cleanly
and efficiently. Exercise lets you keep burning up those
piles of fat even for many hours after a workout. It is
the best way to raise your metabolic rate safely and tell
your body to get rid of that weight which is holding
you back.

Exercise is the solution for those people whose
metabolism is abnormally slow due to genetic factors,
aging, or whatever. Exercise speeds up that slowing
metabolic rate so that they can eat a normal amount
without converting the calories into body fat.

4. *Exercise strengthens you.* As we approach middle age
and beyond, our muscles naturally tend to get weaker.
That lawn mower we could push all morning a few
years ago now seems strangely heavy. That end table
we could easily pick up in our last decade now seems
too unwieldy. Those stairs to the second floor
somehow seem to be twice as high. Regular exercise
won't prevent this decline altogether (it's part of
normal aging), but will slow it down tremendously.
Unless you are completely paralyzed and in a
wheelchair, life makes physical demands on you. You
have to carry in the groceries, run to the bus, or climb
the stairs at work. If you are out of shape, such
activities can strain you and make you huff and puff.
But exercise keeps you strong enough to handle such
activities with a smile.

Once, when I first started getting back into shape as
an adult, my sister-in-law and I had parked the car
and were walking upstairs to a shopping mall. My
sister-in-law, who is thirteen years younger than me,
was groaning and hanging back. It was a steep grade
and she could hardly make it. But I kept walking as if
the path were flat. I didn't even breathe hard!

5. *Exercise makes you healthier.* Our bodies were intended for exercise and work. Lazing around not only weakens your leg and arm muscles, but also the muscles of the organs that keep you alive, particularly the heart and lungs. Believe me, your heart is the most important muscle in your body. If you exercise it well, it will take much better care of you. Active exercise raises the heart rate for a while, but getting into shape lets your heart work less the rest of the day. In other words, your resting pulse rate goes down because your heart pumps with greater vigor and volume of blood per stroke. This keeps your heart stronger and healthier for a longer time.

   H. T., for example, was the hospitalized patient of a doctor who corresponded with me. This guy was in bad shape due to poor diet, lack of exercise, and alcoholism. His heart was so bad that he had to have a quadruple coronary bypass operation. This means that the artery that feeds blood to his heart was in rotten condition, and he was ripe for a deadly heart attack. After his surgery, however, he got on an improved diet and a minimal exercise program. Even with his far-advanced and deadly serious heart condition, he made a miraculous recovery!

   As long as you're alive, it's never too late for an improved diet and exercise program to help you! Never!

6. *Exercise can lengthen your life.* If exercise makes you healthier, it is no surprise that it can lengthen your life. Of course, any of us could die at any time from being hit by a truck or in some other accident. But if you do live until you die of natural causes, this will probably occur later in life if you exercise regularly. (Whatever years you have left will also be filled with more life and a greater sense of physical well-being.)

   One study examined the life habits and death rates of 16,936 Harvard alumni.[1] They found that *any kind of exercise,* including walking and stair climbing as well as sports, *lowered the death rate.* The more the exercise, the lower the death rate, even among people who smoked and were overweight. For those who burned 2000 or more calories *per week* in exercise, the death rate was one-third lower than for those who did not exercise. That many calories is roughly equivalent to jogging or walking about twenty miles per week, or three miles a day (it takes about 100 calories per mile). But even much less exercise than that lengthened life. Among people eighty years old or over, starting an exercise program could add up to two or more years of life on the average. This is an amazingly detailed study, and if exercise alone has such wonderful effects, imagine what exercise combined with a good diet and no smoking can do!

7. *Exercise makes you feel good.* Since exercise makes you healthier, naturally you feel better. As you keep your weight and appetite under control, you also feel more satisfied with yourself. You gain a sense of self-confidence and a radiance that will help you at work and in your social life. You also get what has been called "a runner's high." It seems that the brain produces chemicals called endorphins when you exercise.[2] These chemicals give you a glowing feeling of happiness and even exaltation. Furthermore, regular exercise will usually help you sleep better, which makes you feel more rested during the day. (Just don't exercise within about two hours of going to bed, or the resulting bodily arousal might keep you awake.)

8. *Exercise helps you cope with stress.* With more and more stress in modern life, the best way I know of to deal with it is also the oldest: simple exercise. Somehow, doing an exercise that you like drains away tensions, allows you to think more clearly, and helps you cope better. If you are out of shape and often tense, try this for yourself and see how well it works.

9. *Exercise improves your mental state.* Exercise not only helps you physically, but also psychologically. It seems to clarify the thought processes, boost your mood state, and make you feel on top of the world. One study of sixty middle-aged men who were out of shape found that beginning a simple exercise program quickly made radical changes in them.[3] They grew more emotionally stable, self-confident, and optimistic. A study of seventy men ranging in age from twenty-four to sixty-eight found improvements in their ability to take tests.[4] After only four months in the exercise program, they actually scored higher on certain intelligence tests!

In short, exercise not only helps you with dieting and fat, it helps you with practically all of your life.

What the Bible Says

Proverbs 31:27 tells us that the good wife "does not eat the bread of idleness." Notice how eating is linked with lack of exercise. Idle people have more appetite, even though they're burning fewer calories. But to be idle and to eat more only makes you put on weight.

Proverbs 12:11 says, "He who tills his land will have plenty of bread." Working hard provides you with more food or more of the means to obtain food. Using up stored calories in hard work also makes you better able to enjoy your food. When you work more you can eat more, while still maintaining or losing body weight. So if you eat more of a balanced diet, you'll get more of the valuable nutrients you need.

Second Thessalonians 3:10–12 adds, "If any one will not work, let him not eat. For we hear that some of you are living in idleness, mere busybodies, not doing any work. Now such persons we command and exhort in the Lord Jesus Christ to do their work in quietness and to earn their own living." This passage has many meanings; for instance, it tells how public welfare programs should be run. But I also see here a dietary lesson: If you don't work (exercise), but still eat normally, you are inputting more calories than you output. You are letting yourself slip into the uncomfortable position of adding fat. Instead, you should try to align input/output by balancing exercise with the amount you eat.

Ensuring Enough Exercise

Whenever you exercise, unless it's something moderate like a walk, always stretch and warm up *before* starting. About ten or fifteen minutes is usually enough. Stretching is important because it can help prevent pulled muscles and similar injuries. And after a vigorous exercise session, *always* cool down gradually. Take about ten minutes to stretch and walk it off. The worst thing you can do after a good workout like a fast jog is to stop suddenly and sit or lie down. This puts a terrible strain on your system, and can even be dangerous.

Remember, *always* warm up before a good workout and *always* cool down after one.

If you experiment, you will find the mix between rest and exercise that is right for you. I used to exercise three times a day almost every day. But I found that that made my muscles and joints sore after several days in a row. So I cut back to twice every day and only occasionally take a third outing.

Listen to your body and go at the pace that is right for you. Do *not* try to force yourself to meet the standards of others, the standards you once met when you were younger, or some arbitrary future goals you have set for yourself. Go out and have fun. Do as much as feels good—no more, no less. And watch that fat melt away, to be replaced by firm, lean muscle.

Don't think of exercise as being only planned events where you put on a special uniform and time yourself or compete. In every activity of daily life think of ways to be more rather than less physically active. For example, if my kids want me to take them to the candy store a mile away, I'll do it. But we don't drive and make it a quick hop. We all walk and make a fun trip out of it. Also, when I take the commuter train I get off at the stop before mine and walk the extra mile to and from work.

Here are some more ideas for adding physical activity to your daily life:

How to Be More Physically Active

- Use the stairs rather than the elevator.
- Put more vigor into everyday activities.
- Take several one-minute stretch breaks during the day.
- Take a walk each day at lunchtime or after work.
- Attend an aerobics or slimnastics class.
- Develop a "do it yourself" home exercise program.
- Establish a regular weekly schedule for activities such as swimming or tennis.
- Set up a daily routine of walking, bicycling, or jogging.
- Play basketball in the community gym or your own backyard.
- Join an office, intramural, or community sports league.
- Go dancing or join a square dance club.

Look at your list to see how to best fit "fitness" into your schedule. Then *take action*. But remember, *keeping fit* is an ongoing process. Once you've worked up to a new level of activity, stick with it! When you're ready, increase your activity level even more.

Source: Dietary Guidelines for Americans, U. S. Department of Agriculture: Home and Garden Bulletin Number 232-2 (April, 1986), p. 7.

Special Exercises

To some people calisthenics represents the ultimate terror among exercise activities. I personally don't enjoy them, either. But among my fifteen or sixteen exercise periods a week, I also add about ten minutes of calisthenics to three of them. That's not so much that it bothers me, but it is enough to stretch and strengthen arm, leg, and stomach muscles.

Doing exercises like these, or ones of your own design or from other fitness programs, can help you with weight control and waistline control. Becky is forty-seven years old and married. Since her days in school she has tried just about every popular diet that's blown through the mass media. She stuck faithfully to each in turn, for several days or weeks at a time, and only gained more weight. Then she began to add exercise, as I recommended, and forgot about all the fad diets. In only four months she lost twenty pounds, declining from 155 to 135. She is still on the healthy diet/exercise plan, and still losing!

Carol never needed to diet because she used exercise to keep from ever adding excess fat in the first place. She is now thirty, single, and stands five feet, two inches tall. She works as a sales representative for a pharmaceutical company. At 105 pounds, she has never been on a fad diet because she never needed to lose weight. For her, eating a balanced diet, doing aerobics, and occasionally lifting weights are enough. Not only has she kept slim and muscular, but she adds, "I feel good. I have more energy."

How would you like to duplicate her success?

EXERCISE
ADDS YEARS
TO LIFE
AND
LIFE TO
THE YEARS

14

Diet, Health, and Sex

The GIO-KIO health plan does a number of things for you. It lets you eat all you need, as long as you choose the right foods. It lets you eat anything you want, as long as you restrict amounts of less-healthy items. It reduces your body fat, makes you healthier, and improves how you look and feel.

Is it any wonder, then, that the plan can improve your sex appeal and enjoyment of sensuality?

I'm talking about married people who want to put the zip back into their sex lives. They can make themselves more physically and psychologically attractive, more exciting to their mates. They can enjoy themselves—and each other—as they haven't in decades.

Does this pattern sound familiar? Marriage starts off warm and exciting, then career pressures and the responsibilities of rearing a family come along. Age begins to creep up, slowly at first, but steadily advancing. Bulges start appearing in the wrong places and firm muscles grow lax. Both partners start to feel more blah and worn out in general. When it comes to the bedroom, the first thing they think of is sleep.

There's no way to stop completely the aging process, but diet and exercise can help to slow it down. In terms of your heart, lungs, muscles, waistline, and sense of vigor, you *can* become more like you were ten, fifteen, or even more years ago. In some cases you can become even better! For instance, I can do more push-ups and run farther now than I could twenty years ago.

If you feel fifteen years younger, if you look fifteen years younger, if your body acts fifteen years younger, you will appeal to your partner as if you were fifteen years younger. You can't really turn back the clock, but you can make your body more like it was in your youth. This really works!

Dr. Herbert A. de Vries of the Andrus Gerontology Center at the University of Southern California explored the effects of exercise on the body. People who had been out of shape for decades got into the kind of exercise routine recommended by the GIO-KIO diet and health plan. In a few weeks they dropped body fat, lowered their blood pressure, strengthened their hearts and lungs, and reduced nervous tension. As de Vries put it, they "became as fit and energetic as those twenty to thirty years younger."

I know several couples who clearly demonstrate the truth of this, and the wonderful effect it can have on their sex lives. Ted was only thirty-three years old but he had not engaged in regular exercise for a dozen years. To relax, he watched TV and read rather than jog or play tennis. He was only slightly overweight, but enough out of shape that walking up a flight of stairs quickly got to him. During sexual relations with his wife, he noticed sometimes that his heart seemed to be under a strain. Rather than making him feel elated and joyful, sex sometimes seemed to wear him out completely. He decided to get back into physical shape, if for no other reason than to become a better lover to his wife. He had the doctor check out his heart and it was normal, though rather weak. For exercise, Ted started walking the dog, a little more each time, until he started feeling strong and vigorous again. Even without changing his diet, he also lost a few pounds this way. He could tighten his belt up a notch. And in the bedroom he became a sure and confident lover again.

Betty married at twenty-two and began to grow rotund almost immediately. By twenty-eight she had a major weight problem.

Her husband, who was three years older, retained his slim waist and muscular build. Betty felt ashamed, as if she had somehow betrayed her husband. Though he never complained or said anything unkind about her condition, Betty felt that he must resent the change in her. He must wonder where his slender wife had disappeared. She resolved to lose the excess weight, and she did it. Her husband was delighted to see again the woman he had married. Though his behavior toward her didn't really change, Betty herself did. She felt more attractive, so she *acted* more attractive. She felt more self-confident and secure about her body and expressing her sexual feelings. It was this, rather than the weight loss itself, that reinvigorated their sex life.

Not all of these stories have happy endings. Larry and Sandra both started to gain weight and lose their shapes at about the same time. This didn't particularly bother Sandra, but Larry felt dismayed. He made a pact with his wife that both of them would get back into shape. It would be each partner's gift to the other. Sandra grudgingly agreed, apparently not believing that either would keep this bargain. But Larry stuck with his pact. He consulted physical training experts, joined a gym, worked out with weights, practiced calisthenics, and started jogging. He not only lost all his flab, he put on more muscle than he had had sixteen years previously when in high school. He developed a much keener interest in things physical, including sex. The failure of Sandra to show any improvement at all upset and finally angered him. He reminded her of the pact, cajoled, and pleaded with her. She could not or would not change. This couple had other sources of marital disharmony, and the weight problem didn't help. Perhaps that was the straw that broke the camel's back. In spite of having two young daughters, they separated and ultimately divorced.

The Sexual Benefits of Diet

1. *Weight-loss effects.* A flatter stomach makes you more physically attractive. I once read about a survey that asked a number of women what they found most sexy

about a man. The most common response was a flat stomach. Men have similar reactions about women. Dr. Sherwin A. Kaufman, author of *Sexual Sabotage*, reports that one of the major sexual turnoffs for men is having their wives become overweight.

That may not be fair, but it's a fact. I'm sure none of these respondents meant to put down plumper people in any way. I think we would all agree that human dignity, spiritual maturity, and worth as a person have virtually nothing to do with weight or body size. But what others *think* of you may have a lot to do with just that.

Our concepts of beauty have, of course, been conditioned tremendously by society. We see, for example, fashion models and youthful actors who are almost always slender, muscular, and shapely. That affects our perceptions of sex appeal, whether we want it to or not.

Furthermore, if two partners are both distinctly obese, they may experience some difficulty in the physical aspects of making contact. Overweight does not necessarily make sexual activity impossible, but it can interfere. When overweight people lose the extra poundage, they can engage in more variations of sexual activity than they could before.

2. *Nutritional balance effects.* Fad diets can put a real dent in your sex life while you are on them. If you feel starved and weak all day, if you feel cranky, moody, and irritable because of hunger, you have less desire for sexual activity. It can make you less able or willing to respond if your partner tries to initiate relations.

Like any other part of the body, the sexual organs require balanced nutrition to perform at their best. Sexual hormones, for instance, are chemicals formed in the body from other chemicals that are derived, ultimately, from the foods you eat. A shortage of the required raw materials in your diet may affect the supply of finished chemicals your body can make, as a shortage of lumber could affect the number of houses you could build.

A severely unbalanced diet may lead to impotence or even sterility. Diet can also interact with various diseases that affect sexuality. For instance, diabetes can cause male impotence, but a good diet like the GIO-KIO one, which is low in simple carbohydrates but high in complex ones, can help control diabetes and prevent this effect. Arteriosclerosis (hardening of the arteries) in the pelvic region can also cause impotence, but a diet low in fat and cholesterol can help prevent this from happening. Hypertension (high blood pressure), which can be worsened by excess salt in the diet, can make sex difficult or unsafe. Poor diet may be one of the reasons that 40 percent of men over the age of forty experience some impotence or related problems with sexual performance.[1]

3. *Energy level effects.* It takes energy to conduct any sort of physical activity. It has been estimated that even one kiss of average intensity expends nine calories.[2] (At that rate, if you kissed 389 times you could lose a pound of fat!) All sexual activities burn calories: they not only feel good, they provide exercise that strengthens the whole system. Sex can help you use up excess calories and lose weight. The longer and more frequent your lovemaking sessions, the more calories you use up in this way. Some doctors estimate that you can burn up to about 300 calories in a complete episode of sexual intercourse.

Since sexual activity requires energy, a fad diet that provides low energy can markedly interfere with one's love life. Some conscientious objectors during World War II volunteered to undergo a period of semistarvation so that doctors could study the effects.[3] The study directors wanted to learn more about how they could treat the victims of concentration camps who were being liberated and all the starving refugees produced by the war. These volunteers ended up getting a low-calorie diet that is remarkably like some of the more extreme fad diets of today. For the study they lived in a barracks-type arrangement where their food intake could be controlled and monitored. These young guys normally thought quite a bit about women and sex and would put up pictures of beautiful girls in their lockers and talk and dream about women. But as they lost a lot of weight and experienced serious hunger, all that changed. They started talking and dreaming about food rather than females. They even put pinup pictures of delicious food in their lockers! This complete change in interests seriously affected their relationships with the women in their lives. By the end of the twenty-four-week study, many couples had broken up.

This study demonstrates that fad diets based on severe deprivation can seriously interfere with the normal sex drive, even though they help one to lose weight (temporarily). Simple weight loss at all costs does not provide the answer; but a healthy diet like the GIO-KIO plan *can* help you reverse some of the ravages of time, lose weight, and become more sexy.

The Sexual Benefits of Exercise

1. *Firming the muscles.* Exercise uses your muscles. When an exercise affects a given muscle repeatedly, the muscle responds by growing firmer and stronger. It adds protein and maintains a higher level of muscle tone. On the other hand, failing to use a given muscle on a regular basis leads to its wasting away to a certain extent. Conducting limited exercises that work on only part of the body will help those parts only, not your whole body. For instance, if your only exercise is walking, this will help your leg and back muscles, or those you are actually using. But it will do nothing for your arm muscles. This is why a well-rounded exercise program is important.

Firm, strong muscles make both sexes look more

attractive. Given the same amount of fat in the stomach, for instance, a person with weak stomach and back muscles will bulge out more around the waist. A person with firm stomach muscles will not show his or her fat so much. (It's even better to reduce the fat *and* firm the stomach.)

Firm muscles make a man look more masculine and a woman look more feminine. For a man, a certain amount of bulge in his biceps (arm muscles), pectorals (chest muscles), and quadriceps (thigh muscles) is considered attractive. Women typically don't want those kinds of muscles. But exercise helps them also to retain their distinctively feminine shape.

In short, the *only* way to firm up your muscles is through exercise. And firm muscles make anyone look sexier than he or she does otherwise.

2. *Cardiovascular conditioning.* Any kind of exercise helps strengthen the internal organs like the heart and lungs, organs that must respond to all sorts of physical activity. Running or playing tennis or mowing the lawn can all help increase your physical endurance. Since sexual activity also requires physical endurance, any kind of regular exercise will make a person more capable of sustained and active sexual relations.

As people get older, they often wonder if sex is dangerous for a weak heart. Can sex cause a heart attack? There is no doubt that sex combined with guilt or unusual excitement, usually associated with visiting a prostitute or illicit lover, has occasionally led to a fatal heart attack. However, most people, no matter how old or bad their hearts, can safely engage in sexual relations in the context of a loving, secure marriage. The physical exercise of sex and the resulting emotional gratification can in that case be positively healthy for the heart.

After a heart attack, most doctors do recommend that a couple wait eight to twelve weeks before resuming sexual relations. When the heart attack victim returns to other normal activities, sex may also be resumed. The peak heart rate reached during normal activities like walking up stairs is about 120, while that reached during orgasm is no more than about 117 beats per minute.

3. *Heightened sensory awareness.* Regular exercise puts you more in touch with your own body. You become more aware of your strengths and limitations; you feel more alive, more aware. You feel more in tune with your own senses, better able to respond in a sensuous way, and more easily aroused. The nerves conduct impulses faster, your coordination improves, and you feel less tense and more able to relax and concentrate on your beloved. You are more agile and better able to maneuver. Your joints can bend and move freely.

In short, when it comes to sex, few things can help like a good diet and exercise program. And, in turn, sexual activity can help you lose weight. It not only gives you something else to enjoy rather than more dessert, but it actually burns calories. Diet and exercise can rejuvenate your love life.

A GOOD DIET
AND
REGULAR EXERCISE
MAKES *YOU*
MORE SEXY

———————————

Section IV

Changing Your Life

15

Changing Food Habits

Planning to eat and preparing the right foods are not always enough. To get and stay healthy, you also may need to change some of your eating habits. By giving more attention to this side of your life, you can help control calories and eat properly, thereby aiding your digestion, mood, and health.

Become Aware

Become aware of your eating habits. It may be that you do certain things so mechanically that you don't even realize them. For instance, when and where do you typically note food cravings for salty/sugary/fatty snacks? When watching TV? When conversing on the phone with friends? At parties? If your own behavior is not obvious to you, it may help to keep a log or journal. Alternatively, you might want to ask your spouse, children, other relatives, or friends who know you well what your eating "weaknesses" are.

Self-Examination

Once you realize your habits, examine them closely. Which do you want to keep? Which do you want to get rid of? Think

about this carefully in the context of all you've read in this book.
Pray about it seriously and ask God's guidance. Don't think only
in terms of your stomach size here; rather, think about whether
or not your actions bring glory to God. Are you ashamed of any
of your eating behaviors? Do you help or mislead others by your
example? Particularly with regard to your own children, are you
setting a good example that will help them grow up healthy and
strong? Or are you initiating them into your own bad habits,
setting the stage for them to become overweight or less healthy
in later life? This is the acid test for whether you think a given
habit is positive or negative: Do you want your own children to
pick it up?

Commitment

For habits that you think are unworthy of you, that you want
to change, make a commitment to do so. Write down your goals
on your weight-loss chart or on a separate sheet of paper. For
example, "I *will* stop eating ice cream as a snack. I *will* eat only
one serving per day as a dessert." Or, "I *will* stop eating candy
while watching TV." Remind yourself of these goals every day.
Pray about them. Ask God for guidance on how to meet these
goals and for the power to do it.

Think Positive

Always stress the positive! You must not think of this plan as
deprivation, as giving up things you like. First, you should only
make changes because they will help you. They will make you
thinner, healthier, and happier. You are making these changes
because you see a greater good ahead. Second, if you give up
something, don't leave a void. Whenever possible, practice
replacement rather than simple denial. For instance, if for years
you have munched on candy while watching TV, you may find
it hard to simply stop eating altogether. Shift to butterless
popcorn at such times. Or shift to a healthy vegetable snack like
plain celery and carrot sticks. As you start making changes, I

don't want you to see a dark tunnel ahead, but rather the light at the end.

Right now as you consider changes, you may feel dread at the idea of leaving behind your bondage to bad habits. You may experience some uncertainty as you move into the desert of change. But if you stick with it, you will soon enter the promised land of health and plenty—and it won't take you forty years, either! You will notice amazing improvements in your mood, sense of well-being, and energy level within twenty-four hours after starting Daniel's ten-day diet challenge and the GIO-KIO diet and health plan. Many people notice marked improvements *even in the first hour* after their first healthy meal! And within one to three days, you will notice the needle on your bathroom scale going down.

By then, you will not see this plan as giving up good things. Once you're safely in the promised land of good eating, *you will not want to go back to your old habits*. You'll be too happy where you are to look back. You will not feel imprisoned by the plan, but free from bad dietary habits for the first time in your life!

Keep Reviewing the Plan

Remind yourself frequently of the key principles of the GIO-KIO plan. Go back and reread key chapters, particularly chapter 5, or return to this summary here. The basic ideas of the plan are as follows:

1. Too much rich food can ruin your health and cut years or even decades off your life. It can take a lot of the life out of your years.
2. Being overweight, regardless of cause, can increase your chances of dying at every age. It can ruin your self-image and social life.
3. It is the responsibility of those who believe God created them to protect that creation. Developing better eating habits can help do just that.

4. Food is not an enemy. God created our bodies and designed food that would meet our bodily needs in the best way possible. We can enjoy food as long as we approach it the way God designed it.

5. Learn to listen to and trust the hunger signal and satiation system that God built in. Whenever you're hungry, eat; snack whenever you want. *You can eat all you want as long as you choose the right foods.* And you can eat anything you want as long as you restrict amounts of the less healthy items. You will *still* lose weight and increase health because you will have learned to trust not only the hunger start-eating system, but also the satiation stop-eating system. In other words, when you are no longer hungry, you'll stop eating or avoid eating in the first place. You won't eat for emotional reasons or recreation, but only when your body says it needs food.

6. The most important single dietary change you can make is to reduce your intake of fats, especially animal fats. This means getting rid of visible fat, reducing your intake of foods with high levels of built-in fat, and not cooking with fat. It takes fat to make fat. Reducing dietary fat will make your own body fat melt away and introduce you to new levels of glowing health.

7. The second most important dietary change you can make is to reduce your intake of processed sugars. Instead, enjoy sweets mostly as God designed them— eat lots of fresh fruit and sweet vegetables.

8. Avoid excess protein in the diet. Particularly, cut down on meat, which is usually high in fat and cholesterol. Two small servings a day of high-protein foods is enough.

9. Reduce salt in your diet whenever possible, especially if you are or anyone in your family is prone to high blood pressure. Cut down not only on use of the salt shaker while cooking and at the table, but also on all condiments and foods high in salt, particularly salty snacks.

10. Eat a variety of whole, fresh, natural foods that are high in complex carbohydrates, particularly whole-grain cereals, fruits, and vegetables. Get some meat, dairy products, and nuts, but not too much.

11. Drink PLENTY of water, at least two to three quarts a day. Whenever possible, drink fresh, plain water rather than high-calorie, caffeine-containing, or other flavored beverages. (*Exception:* Some fruit juice and milk are good every day.) This will not only cut down on calories and possibly unhealthy chemicals, but it will save money in your food budget. Drinking plenty of water before and during meals helps you feel full before you eat too much solid food.

12. Find exercises you like and do them for at least twenty to thirty minutes at a time, at least three days a week. Become more active in doing your work, household chores, and other functions of daily living.

13. A good diet and exercise can make you look and feel younger. They can make you more sexy, and sexual activity can help you exercise and lose weight.

14. Replace bad food habits with healthy ones.

Listen to Your Body

Eat whenever you're hungry, but stop before you feel completely full. Within fifteen to thirty minutes, you will feel full even without eating any more. It takes that much time for the hunger/satiation system to catch up with how much you've been chowing down. When you're not hungry, don't eat, no matter what anyone else (except your doctor) says.

Watch Eating Speed

Try to eat more slowly. There are many reasons for this:

1. When you eat too fast, you tend to eat too much. You pack food in faster than your system can evaluate it and tell you you've eaten enough. Eating more slowly

allows your hunger-satiation system to catch up with how much you're chowing down.

2. You enjoy dining more. The experience of a meal or snack lasts longer, making it seem as if you've eaten more. This way you get more of a chance to notice and savor the different tastes and textures of your food.

3. Slow eating tremendously aids digestion. Have you ever been stressed, in a big hurry, and gulped down your meal? You probably had stomach cramps and indigestion afterward. Chewing more slowly and more thoroughly allows your teeth to grind up the food better, mix it more completely with saliva, and prepare it more properly for the stomach. Otherwise, you send the load down to your stomach unprepared and force the rest of your system to deal with an overload of work. Think of an assembly line in which the first guy doesn't do his job right; that makes it worse for everybody else down the line.

Don't Mix Activities

Don't try to eat while doing anything but socializing. Don't exercise, work, drive, bathe, or watch TV. Many people like to have their meals while watching TV. As long as you don't overeat, there's no real harm in having a healthful snack while watching the tube. But if you eat whole meals that way, you're robbing yourself of the chance to socialize with family or friends. And you're distracting yourself from enjoying your food. Worse, the linking of TV with eating gives you a powerful temptation to overeat: You "feel hungry" not when your body needs food, but when you turn on the glowing box.

If you fall into this category, you need to *break the habit connection between TV and eating.* Don't watch TV while eating, and don't eat while watching TV. Keep these two parts of your life separate. If it helps you to make the transition from current habit linkage to this separation, shift first to eating only healthful snacks while watching the tube.

Avoid Convenience Foods

As a general rule, "convenience" foods, or fully prepared foods, save you time. But they usually cost more and are less healthy than their natural counterparts. They usually have too much salt, sugar, and fat. Even worse, they make eating and snacking too easy. The temptation to rip open a bag of chips can become irresistible.

That is, if you keep such stuff in the house. You may experience some difficulty in shifting from your current habits to avoiding prepared snack foods, but start making the effort. Buy less and less of this stuff. If you have it at home, keep it out of sight, hidden behind more healthy items.

But as I've stressed again and again, don't deprive yourself. If you feel a genuine hunger or even a snack craving, by all means get yourself something to eat. But start first with a healthy, fresh vegetable or fruit. Get something that's good for you. And choose something that you have to get up and fix, for example, to wash and to peel. If you have to expend even that much effort, as opposed to opening a box of cookies, you will automatically think twice whether you are truly hungry or reaching for a snack out of habit.

Menu Planning

Each day plan out your meals and snacks fairly carefully to ensure that you get the right balance of foods as discussed in chapter 5. Think in long-range terms when you do your grocery shopping to ensure that you purchase enough variety and quantity of items. Always go grocery shopping right after you have eaten so that you buy what you plan to buy and are not led astray by hunger and cravings. (Try to avoid the junk food aisles altogether.)

Once you know what foods to eat, then you don't worry about how much. You don't have to measure and restrict portion sizes (except for desserts and the high-fat foods you're trying to cut down on). You don't have to count calories. You can eat *all* you want of the healthy, balanced, fresh foods like whole-grain cereal products, fruits, and vegetables.

In Appendix A I've provided an exhaustive table that gives the calorie values of virtually all common foods. This is not for you to start researching all your meals and then scribble away numbers and compute totals. Instead, note which foods are grouped together so that you can make substitutions as desired to introduce more variety into your diet. For example, use the list to remind you of the great variety of fruits that are available. Then select a different combination of fruits whenever you go to the grocery store.

Second, I want you to have this list so you can check out which foods are higher in calories than others. Generally, these are the higher-fat items that you want to minimize.

You can eat your fill of the lower-fat and lower-calorie items. You will *not* suffer hunger, but you *will* lose weight on the GIO-KIO plan. You will get more balanced nutrition than you do now, and you will soon, very soon, start to look and feel better. Medical tests that your doctor uses to assess the state of your health will prove that these changes are not just in your mind. Your blood cholesterol and triglyceride (fat) levels will go down. All your standard laboratory tests of blood and urine should show improvement.

My own blood test a few weeks after I took Daniel's ten-day diet challenge and modified my diet showed a healthy drop of thirty-three points, from a reading of 198 to one of 165, which is clearly on the positive side of the scale (cholesterol over 200 to 220 starts to get dangerous, as was reported in chapter 1).

What better reward could there be for changed eating habits? That you will soon be buying new clothes with smaller waist sizes should also help.

Add Less Salt and High-Calorie Condiments

I remember when I was a kid how much I liked chocolate sundaes. I would eat great oozing piles of chocolate syrup one day, and want more the next. It became like a drug: I needed more each successive time to tease my jaded taste buds. Finally I realized what was happening and quit regular use of chocolate syrup altogether. For decades, I have used it only on infrequent, special occasions.

The trouble with added salt, sugar, fat (cooking oil, mayonnaise, salad dressing, etc.), and other condiments is that the more you get, the more you want. If you add 200 milligrams of salt to your popcorn one day, you'll want 205 the next, and 210 the day after, and so on. If salt has lost its savor for you, throw it out (Matthew 5:13). That is, get rid of the salt shaker and quit using added salt.

Yet, oddly enough, once you start cutting down on these condiments, you'll enjoy natural foods more. You'll uncover the fresh, original tastes that you had long forgotten. You'll feel as if you've gone to another country and discovered an entirely new menu. You'll get there faster if you cut out such condiments cold turkey. If that thought alarms you or upsets your appetite, then cut down gradually to the point where you're adding the least you can get away with and still enjoying your food.

At the same time that you enjoy your diet all the more, you'll be protecting your body from the adverse effects of these condiments in excess.

Eating Out Wisely

It's relatively easy to plan your own diet when you're eating at home. But often you want or need to eat out. That can pose problems but if you're careful, you'll be all right. It may be that you eat out so rarely (once a week or less) that you'd like that to be your splurge time. You don't want to worry about selecting the right foods then. You'd rather enjoy the not-so-healthy foods you've been cutting down on the rest of the week. I think that's a viable option, so long as you don't overdo it. Once your body has adjusted to less salt, sugar, and fat, if you go back suddenly to the amounts you used to consume, you will really overload your system.

Be careful! If you used to eat twenty-one-ounce steaks, but for the last month have eaten no more than five ounces of meat a day, your body has adjusted to that change. A nine-ounce steak will seem like as much a splurge to you now as the larger one once did. The twenty-one-ounce job would place a strain on your system, so much so that I don't think you would enjoy the last half of it.

If you choose not to splurge but stick to the GIO-KIO plan as a rule when eating out, I think that is preferable, especially if you must eat out often. You don't want to undo in five or seven meals a week everything you've worked so hard to do in the remaining ones.

When eating out, therefore, I suggest you generally avoid dishes high in meat, sauce, and gravy. Start with a fruit cup or tossed salad with little or no regular dressing. (If they don't have low-cal dressing, ask for vinegar and a sprinkle of herb mix, or something similar.) Order several vegetables or a vegetarian platter. Have a baked potato rather than French fries (fried in fat) or mashed potatoes with gravy. Use sour cream rather than butter on your potato. Stick to seafood rather than large, fatty meat entrees. Ask for broiled rather than fried, breaded, and deep-fried items. For dessert select something fresh and cool, like fruit or jello, rather than a hypersweet and fatty-rich item.

I don't mean to sound heartless, as if you're supposed to give up all your favorite treats. I am only suggesting the maximally beneficial items in each category (appetizer, entree, side dishes, and dessert). You're supposed to enjoy food; the whole point of going out to eat usually is to enjoy yourself. Instead of splurging in every category, just splurge in one or two. For instance, make sure you get a good balance for the rest of your meal, and then go ahead and have a slice of Boston cream pie or German chocolate cake.

Weighing Yourself

Don't weigh yourself too often. If you weigh yourself every day—or, even worse, more frequently—you will confuse your true loss of fat with normal up and down changes in weight due to salt, water retention, waste retention, time of day, and so on. For the same reason, weigh yourself at the same time of day and under the same conditions whenever you do so. For example, if you weigh yourself right after dinner, you may grow disappointed to see your weight is the same as last week, if at that time you weighed yourself right after a jog and before breakfast.

Your weight can easily fluctuate as much as a pound or two over the hours of any one day. But little of that change is due to alterations in the amount of fat. Most of it is water. I recommend that you weigh yourself only once a week at most. If you follow the GIO-KIO plan closely, but don't push yourself into serious hunger, you will lose between one and two pounds a week in real fat. In the early stages of the diet, you may also lose some body water that was held in place by excess salt. So your scale weight may go down even faster than two pounds a week at first. Write down your weight each week on the Weight Loss Chart (Appendix B) so you can keep track of your progress.

If you press yourself into serious hunger or exercise drastically, *which I do* not *recommend*, you may show faster initial losses. But you may also get sick of the diet that way, go off it, and rebound into gaining back all your lost weight.

Remember, the GIO-KIO plan is a complete diet and health plan that you can live with for the rest of your life! Don't get into such a hurry at first that you burn out. It's not how you start the race against fat, but how you finish it that counts.

Depending on how much extra fat you start with, it may take you few or a number of weeks to reach your goal. As you approach the natural weight that is right for your body composition and build (as determined by your genetic makeup), your weight loss may slow down. If you are losing less than a pound of fat a week, I recommend that you measure your weight less frequently than once a week. In other words, measure it only once every two weeks, or even once a month.

Ideally, you wouldn't need to weigh yourself at all. You would stop worrying about numbers and enjoy the new you emerging in the mirror and fitting into slimmer clothes and a tighter belt. But Americans and people in other advanced societies are obsessed with numbers. So if you are only satisfied with progress if it has a number on it, go ahead and measure it that way.

When your body weight stabilizes for a month, and you are still following the GIO-KIO plan closely, then that probably tells you your natural, ideal body weight. Don't worry if it falls a little lower or higher than your original goal weight. Sometimes your inner body wisdom is greater than your mental knowledge. In that case adjust your goal concepts accordingly.

One reason your actual body weight may stabilize a little above your goal body weight is that you're putting on more muscle. If you get into a serious exercise program as I recommend, you will definitely put on several pounds of muscle over the next few months. Although this will lower the difference between your starting and ending weights, *don't worry about it.* You are still losing fat, but are replacing it with some muscle, muscle that will make you look better and more shapely. It will help you look thin by holding all your body parts in place. It will help keep you vigorous and healthy, for some of the increase in weight will be in your heart and other internal muscles that maintain your vital life functions.

If you have any doubt as to whether you are still carrying too much fat as well, go back to chapter 2 and retry some of those tests for being overweight. If your weight now is mostly muscle, that won't show up in signs of flab.

Watch Out for Alcohol

I've seen well-intentioned Christians and Bible scholars argue a lot about this one. Some point out that God created wine to "gladden the heart of man" (Psalms 104:15). Others counter that grape juice, rather than an alcoholic beverage, is referred to in this and similar verses. What virtually all agree on is that *excess* alcohol is bad. "And do not get drunk with wine . . . but be filled with the [Holy] Spirit" (Ephesians 5:18). I don't want to get involved in a theological discussion of whether or not you should drink alcoholic beverages. But if you do drink, I want you to know the nutritional facts.

Alcohol is the second most concentrated source of calories in the food supply. Fat provides about 255 calories per ounce, and alcohol about 200, whereas protein and carbohydrates only yield about 113. If you drink a lot, therefore, you will greatly increase your calorie load and your chances of growing and staying fat.

Furthermore, alcohol provides nothing more nutritional than simple energy. It can be used by the body only for energy; it neither helps build nor maintain bodily tissues. Certain beverages like beer, of course, contain more than alcohol. Beer also has lots of water, some carbohydrate, a little protein, and small amounts of several vitamins and minerals. However, there are far more important and richer sources of these nutrients than beer. And they usually come with fewer calories.

For instance, a single slice of whole-wheat bread has about half the calories of a bottle of beer, the same carbohydrate, three times the protein, ten times the iron, and more of most of the other minerals and vitamins. On balance then, beer does provide some nutrition, but less than most other sources.

However, wines contain even fewer nutrients, and whiskeys practically none. Remember, alcohol itself provides no nutrition other than energy. So, insofar as it replaces more healthful foods in the diet, alcohol impedes nutrition. Furthermore, alcohol in excess interferes with absorption of many of the nutrients that you're taking in from the other foods you eat.[1] Excess alcohol interferes with intestinal absorption of the vitamins thiamin, niacin, B_6, and B_{12}.

These nutrients are all important for health. It should come as no surprise then that alcoholism is associated with such diseases as anemia, cirrhosis of the liver (one of the leading causes of death), hypoglycemia, and pancreatitis, among others.[2]

Alcohol affects the physical structure of the cellular membranes in many different organs.[3] It can actually damage the protein and lipid components of the cell walls. Thus in excess it can poison and even kill cells in such organs as the brain, heart, and pancreas, as well as liver.

If you do drink, *do not drink to excess*. Most authorities recommend no more than two drinks per day, or the equivalent of no more than an ounce of pure alcohol per day. If you need more specific advice, check with your doctor.

Watch Out for Caffeine

Some people can't get going without their regular infusions of coffee or tea. They are relying on the stimulant compound *caffeine* in such beverages to keep them awake and active. If you feel you must drink caffeine to stay alert, I recommend at least that you cut your intake to half of your usual, and do it immediately. Try to reduce further over the next few weeks.

Caffeine is an addictive drug and after years of drinking it, you seem to need it more as a way of avoiding withdrawal symptoms than of actually enhancing effectiveness. It seems to do the latter mostly among people who are not used to it. In other words, in the beginning of the addiction, it truly gives you a lift above normal; but later, it just prevents a drop below normal. I think you are better off without it except for occasional use, under unusual circumstances that require greater-than-normal alertness (as when you have a long drive, for instance).

Unfortunately, it can be difficult to cut down on caffeine, because it is so prevalent in the food supply. It is found not only in the obvious beverages like coffee and tea, but also in a wide array of cola-type drinks, where it is often added artificially. Most of the caffeine found in soft drinks is that removed during the decaffeination of coffee and then added to these other products.[4] Therefore, I recommend shifting to the caffeine-free alternatives to most of these drinks.

But caffeine is even more widespread than that. It or a related compound appears naturally in a number of foods like chocolate and in a number of medications like diuretics, cold remedies, weight-control aids, and even some aspirin-type pain relievers.[5] (It is not found in plain, pure aspirin, however.)

Excessive caffeine on a regular basis can alter your normal cycles of mood, alertness, and relaxation. If you take it any time after late afternoon, it can interfere with falling asleep even hours later that night.

Worse still, heavy use of coffee in particular has been scientifically associated with a number of medical problems.[6] These include the following:

- *Ulcers.* Coffee irritates the stomach lining and increases the production of stomach acids.
- *Heart attack.* Some studies indicate that the more coffee you drink, the greater your chances of a heart attack. (Other studies disagree, however.)[7]
- *Cancer.* Some studies suggest that lots of coffee can lead to increased risk of such cancers as bladder and breast. (Again, however, other studies disagree.)
- *Birth defects.* Animal studies reveal that high doses of coffee can result in birth defects. Human data are less clear, but it is probably wise for expectant mothers to practice moderation in coffee as in all things.

I recommend that you reduce your intake of caffeine as much as you can and as soon as you can. Until we know more fully about the dangers, that's the wisest course. Meanwhile, I think you will find a low-caffeine or caffeine-free existence makes you feel more relaxed and happy, better able to calm down, rest, and sleep so that you won't be so tired the next day and need another dose.

One of my relatives had a bad reaction to caffeine for years, and didn't even realize that was the reason at first. An annual physical exam revealed an irregular heartbeat, so the doctor questioned her about caffeine intake. She reported that she drank only one cup of coffee a day, which led her to believe that she ingested little caffeine. But the doctor's further questions revealed that she also consumed quite a bit of tea, cola, and chocolate, all of which contain substantial amounts of caffeine.

The doctor had her eliminate all these sources of the drug, and by the next week, the number of extra heartbeats per minute declined by one-half. Two weeks more without caffeine, and her heartbeat was completely back to normal! Not all people are this affected by caffeine, but some certainly are.

Don't Char Your Food

When charbroiling steaks or other meat, when searing meat in a fry pan, when roasting beef and other foods, do not overcook. Some people like their meat well done, but they should cook it no further than the point of looking brown. Any parts of meat or other fats that are charred dark brown or black should be trimmed off and discarded. Such pure-black parts contain carbon residues that have been shown to cause cancer.[8] No one knows the exact amount that is dangerous, but be safe and avoid it completely.

Reward Yourself for Improvements

Many of your most valuable rewards for sticking to the GIO-KIO plan will come automatically. Every time you look in the mirror or see the bathroom scale dip another pound, you will be thrilled with the emerging new you. People will soon notice the difference and praise you for it.

But you can also reward yourself deliberately for showing willpower and restraint, for approaching food more as God would have you do. Make a mental list of special things you like to do: go shopping, take a walk in the park, buy a new magazine. Every now and then, at least once a week, give yourself some special treat. And don't forget to brag to yourself with a little positive self-talk, too. Take pride in your body and in your dietary achievements.

Pray

Don't ever forget that God made you and God made food. There's no one on earth who understands the right connection between the two as well as He does. He's your Father and He will help you understand the proper approach. But you need to ask Him!

Ask God daily for guidance. And ask Him daily for the power you need to handle your food temptations and decisions that day.

IMPROVE
YOUR EATING HABITS
AND
TRANSFORM YOUR LIFE

16

Menus for Daniel's Ten-Day Diet Challenge

Here's your chance to prove to yourself that the typical modern eating habits to which all of us are exposed and to which most of us give in aren't healthy. This is not just a matter of believing scientific studies and textbooks you've read; this is something you will see and feel in your own mind and body, starting almost immediately. You will *know* that the biblical plan for healthy eating, as God designed, works and that it matches your bodily needs.

This is not a matter of wish fulfillment, positive thinking, or delusion. This is *real!* To use a parallel, let's say your car should run on high-octane unleaded fuel. Someone tells you that's too expensive—you should just fill 'er up with a mixture of alcohol and oil. Wouldn't you argue that your car runs better on the fuel for which it was designed? Then this devil's advocate says you only *think* it runs better on unleaded gasoline because you want it to, but really the other mixture is just as good. But it's not that subjective, is it? Couldn't you prove in performance that real gasoline works better than this other "fad fuel"?

If you take Daniel's ten-day diet challenge, you will begin to feel better within hours of your first healthy meal. You will feel stronger, more vigorous, and more alert. You will sleep better. Within a couple of days you will notice the fat disappearing and your clothes feeling looser. Within a week people will begin to notice the difference in you and comment favorably on it.

This is not just in your mind. The bathroom scale doesn't lie; it will show the weight go down. The mirror doesn't lie; it will show that fat slipping away. And if you want some actual proof, let your doctor analyze a sample of your blood before and after you take Daniel's ten-day diet challenge. Remember, I personally compared my cholesterol level before and about two months after starting the diet. My cholesterol level dropped thirty-three points, from 198 to 165, from borderline okay to super healthy! You will no doubt see similar changes in a host of physical measures, if you take them.

Here is the challenge: Follow this pattern for only ten days, as Daniel did in the royal court in Babylon. You don't have to go beyond ten days, for that is enough to prove the superiority of the biblical plan to your old habits. Afterward, you make as many of the right changes in your old habits as you can live with.

We don't know from Scripture the exact foods Daniel chose, or how much he ate. But the same basic principle of selecting only the healthy items from the luxurious diet surrounding him applies today. In the ten days of his diet challenge, he ate only vegetables and water. Later, when he had more control over his menu and food preparation, he added meat and probably other items as well.

The ten-day diet I'm offering here, then, is not copied from a blueprint in the Bible. But it stays true to the spirit of Daniel's challenge: You stick to the healthiest items you can find in whatever situation you are in. Whenever possible, you eat whole, fresh foods as God designed them, not as some marketing executive in a food company decided to alter them.

I've combined in one ten-day period both phases of Daniel's diet. The first three days and Day 8 are strictly vegetarian, with no meat or fish (though animal milk and eggs are retained). If you wish to strictly follow Daniel's pattern, you can rotate through these first three days and Day 8 again and again for a total of ten days. But remember, Daniel chose that stricter phase when he was a captive and had little control over the food brought to him. I think you will find it more comfortable and enjoyable to shift on Day 4 to Daniel's less strict phase in which he added meat.

For these ten days note the following rules, keeping in mind you *do not* have to follow these rules strictly for the rest of your life. Follow them for the first ten days, so you can get the maximum possible difference from your past diet and make a clear comparison. After the ten days, evaluate for yourself which rules you can tolerate and which you can't, though you should be as strict as you can throughout your weight-loss phase, however long that may take.

Later, for your weight-maintenance phase, you can loosen up a bit more. But if you return to all your old dietary habits, you will probably gain back all the weight you lost. You will stay happier and healthier and thinner the closer you stick to this plan. In other words, it is better to stick even to a part of the plan *for the rest of your life* than to stick to all of the plan for only a short while and then give it all up.

Therefore, after the ten days are up, I recommend that you follow the basic structure of the GIO-KIO plan for as long as you can. To introduce more variety, make sensible substitutions for the items listed here. For instance, change from one fruit or vegetable or grain product to another. To make these substitutions, all you need to do is consult the comprehensive lists of foods, organized by type in Appendix A.

I have purposely avoided using trade-name food products for these menus. One way you might wish to introduce more variety after the first ten days is to experiment with various brand-name items, so long as they fit the low-fat, low-sugar, low-salt profile. I refer frequently to the generic "whole-wheat bread." You may find five or ten different brands that you like and want to rotate through to offer yourself more variety.

Here are the rules *for the first ten days:*

1. Cut out all butter, margarine, oil, sugar, salt, mayon-naise, jelly, jam, and other condiments you can feel comfortable with losing. Cut out all coffee, tea, other

caffeinated drinks, and alcoholic beverages you can do without.

2. You can eat less than what is listed, but don't substitute items unless you are *sure* that they have no more fat, protein, sugar, and salt than those listed here.

3. Do not eat more than the amount suggested. Don't try to "cheat" by fudging your measurements. For instance, a rounded tablespoon of butter may contain twice as much as a level one. If you still feel hungry after a meal, wait fifteen to thirty minutes. If the hunger doesn't pass, then eat one of the *free, unlimited* snacks on the menu or have a second helping of the unrestricted items on the menu.

4. Items that are underlined are unrestricted. *You can eat all of these you want.* Don't worry about measuring portion sizes or counting calories.

5. You can eat low-calorie snacks *any time* you feel hungry. For each day's menu, two snacks are listed, one between breakfast and lunch, and one between lunch and dinner. You may, however, eat them at any time you wish. If you can, however, avoid eating two or three hours before you go to bed.

6. You can also eat all you want of the low-calorie snack foods listed in chapter 5 at any time.

7. If you stick closely to the plan, you are allowed one special treat each day. This treat should be eaten as your dessert for the evening meal. Eat it while you are maximally full from dinner. *You can choose any treat you want,* but restrict the amount to no more than 200 calories. Consult the calorie chart in Appendix A to measure the right quantity. For your treats, you *do* need to measure carefully and count calories. This rule applies *only* to your treats.

8. If you are in reasonable physical condition and have been cleared by your doctor, start and maintain your new exercise program throughout these ten days. But start slowly and work your way up gradually. It takes months to get back into shape, not just ten days.

9. Don't weigh yourself too frequently and risk discouragement. Do weigh yourself the morning that you start your program (Day 1), on the morning halfway through (Day 6), and the morning after the end (Day 11). Depending on your current weight and your usual dietary habits, you should lose three to four pounds in ten days. You may lose several additional pounds from your scale weight, but most will be due to water loss.

10. In addition to weighing yourself, note how much better you feel, starting almost immediately. Be sure to write down a brief description of your new sense of vigor, energy, and alertness. Tell your family and close friends what a miraculous improvement has occurred. This may encourage them to get on the diet with you, and you can support one another as you all discover new plateaus of health and happiness.

(*Note:* Menus are listed first; GIO-KIO recipes follow.)

Day 1

***

Breakfast:
Any bran-type cereal, added wheat germ, a slice of whole-wheat toast, a quarter cantaloupe, one cup skim milk.

Snack (optional):
Carrot and celery sticks

Lunch:
Cheese sandwich (whole-wheat bread, one ounce or slice of cheese, lettuce, and tomato), water or diet soda, apple.

Snack:
Grapes or cherries

Dinner:

GIO-KIO Salad, one slice of whole-wheat bread or toast, one bowl of beans and rice, optional treat, water or diet soda.

Day 2

Breakfast:

Unsweetened fruit juice, one egg (boiled or fried with no-stick soybean oil spray rather than butter), one slice whole-wheat toast.

Snack:

Bran muffin.

Lunch:

One bowl of tomato or vegetarian soup, one slice of whole-wheat bread or toast, one cup low-fat yogurt, fresh orange, water or diet soda.

Snack:

One ounce unsalted nuts, dill pickles.

Dinner:

GIO-KIO Salad, one whole-wheat roll or handful of whole-wheat crackers, one cup skim milk, one-half grapefruit, optional treat.

Day 3

Breakfast:

Regular oatmeal (not instant), one cup skim milk, a handful of rye crackers, one-quarter fresh melon.

Snack:

Tomato with one slice cheese.

Lunch:
One bowl of GIO-KIO Bean Casserole, one whole-wheat muffin or roll, water or diet soda, one apple.

Snack:
Blueberries, cranberries, or strawberries.

Dinner:
GIO-KIO Vegetable Stir-Fry, whole-wheat bread or toast, half bowl of black-eyed peas or beans, water or diet soda, treat.

Day 4

Breakfast:
Whole-grain cereal, added wheat germ, one cup skim milk, one whole-wheat muffin or slice of bread, one-half grapefruit.

Snack:
Carrot and celery sticks.

Lunch:
Three ounces of canned sardines or tuna (packed in water), one slice of whole-wheat bread, lettuce, and one-half tomato (sliced), diet soda, one apple.

Snack:
One ounce unsalted nuts or seeds.

Dinner:
GIO-KIO Salad, one baked potato with GIO-KIO Topping, one whole-wheat muffin or handful of crackers, one cup skim milk, one-quarter melon or one-half cup of berries, treat.

Day 5

Breakfast:
Bran cereal, added wheat germ, one cup skim milk, one slice whole-wheat toast, one-quarter melon.

Snack:
Two small graham crackers.

Lunch:
One bowl of cream of mushroom or chicken soup, one whole-wheat muffin or handful of crackers, water or soda, one chilled but fresh peach or nectarine.

Snack:
Unbuttered popcorn, slightly salted if you wish.

Dinner:
GIO-KIO Salad, three ounces lean roast beef or steak, one whole-wheat roll or bread slice, water or diet soda, GIO-KIO Fruit Dessert, treat.

Day 6

Breakfast:
Unsweetened fruit juice, one egg (soft-boiled or poached), whole-wheat toast, apricots or prunes.

Snack:
Raw broccoli and cauliflower, with GIO-KIO Topping as a dip.

Lunch:
GIO-KIO Sandwich, one cup of low-fat yogurt, water or diet soda, one-half cup of grapes or berries.

Snack:
Apple.

Dinner:
GIO-KIO Vegetable Stir-Fry, macaroni and cheese, one whole-wheat roll or muffin, water or diet soda, treat.

Day 7

Breakfast:
Regular oatmeal, one cup skim milk, one bran muffin, one-quarter cantaloupe.

Snack:
Dill pickle and two wheat crackers.

Lunch:
One bowl of chicken noodle or rice soup, one slice of whole-wheat toast, one cup of low-fat yogurt, water or diet soda, one orange.

Snack:
Carrot and celery sticks.

Dinner:
GIO-KIO Salad, three ounces of plain broiled fish, one baked potato with GIO-KIO Topping, water or diet soda, one-half cup of cherries or berries, treat.

Day 8

Breakfast:
Cooked cereal, added wheat germ, one cup skim milk, one slice whole-wheat toast, one fresh pear or one-quarter pineapple.

Snack:
One small packet of raisins.

Lunch:
One bowl of beans and rice, cheese toast (one slice of cheese), water or diet soda, one tangerine or orange.

Snack:
Unbuttered popcorn.

Dinner:
GIO-KIO Salad, one bowl green pea soup, a handful of whole-wheat crackers, GIO-KIO Eggplant Supreme, water or diet soda, treat.

Day 9

Breakfast:
Bran cereal, added wheat germ, one cup skim milk, one-half grapefruit, one whole-wheat English muffin or bagel.

Snack:
Bouillon and whole-wheat crackers.

Lunch:
GIO-KIO Sandwich, tomato juice, one cup yogurt, one apple.

Snack:
Gelatin made with artificial sweetener.

Dinner:
GIO-KIO Salad, one whole-wheat roll or biscuit, GIO-KIO Pasta, one-half cup fresh berries, water or diet soda, treat.

Day 10

Breakfast:
Whole-wheat cereal, added wheat germ, one cup skim milk, one slice whole-wheat toast, one peach or nectarine.

Snack:
One ounce unsalted nuts or seeds.

Lunch:
GIO-KIO Salad, cheese toast (one slice of cheese), water or diet soda, one slice of pineapple or watermelon.

Snack:
Broccoli and cauliflower with GIO-KIO Topping as a dip.

Dinner:
One bowl of onion soup, broiled scallops, shrimp, or other seafood (three ounces only), one baked potato with GIO-KIO Topping, lettuce and tomato, water or diet soda, treat.

GIO-KIO Salad

Include at least five of the following: alfalfa sprouts, bean sprouts, broccoli, cabbage, carrots, cauliflower, celery, cucumbers, greens, kale, lettuce, mushrooms, onions, parsley, peppers, radishes, squash, spinach, tomatoes, watercress, and zucchini. All ingredients should be raw and fresh. From day to day you can vary the composition of the salad by changing the ingredients. This gives you more variety and a better balance. Avoid salad dressings except small amounts of low-calorie ones like GIO-KIO French Dressing. Try vinegar, lemon juice, or a sprinkle of an herb mix instead.

GIO-KIO French Dressing

Yields about one cup. Only ten calories per tablespoon, with no cholesterol or fat. Mix 1½ tablespoons of cornstarch and 2 tablespoons of sugar in a saucepan. Stir in 1 cup water. Cook over low heat until thickened, stirring continuously. Cool slightly, then add ¼ cup vinegar, ¼ teaspoon salt, ½ teaspoon dry mustard, ½ teaspoon paprika, ⅛ teaspoon onion powder, and a sprinkle of garlic powder. Mix thoroughly and store in the refrigerator.

GIO-KIO Bean Casserole

Add 1 cup soaked navy beans, 1 cup rice, 4 medium potatoes (cubed), 1 can stewed tomatoes, 2 medium onions sliced, a little salt and garlic salt. Mix in a large pot, bring to a boil, and then simmer until beans are tender (takes about 3 hours).

GIO-KIO Vegetable Stir-Fry

Heat two teaspoons of oil (preferably safflower) in a fry pan. Add one-half cup each of sliced fresh mushrooms, onions, and any four of your favorite vegetables, sliced or diced. Stir over moderate heat for about four minutes. Mix in 1 tablespoon water and ¼ teaspoon soy sauce, cover, and cook a few more minutes, till tender and crisp.

GIO-KIO Topping

By the tablespoon, butter gives you 100 calories, sour cream 25, and this topping only 10. And it's so easy to make! Mix 1 cup low-fat cottage cheese, 1 tablespoon skim milk, and 2 tablespoons lemon juice in a blender. Whip until the mixture is smooth and creamy. Serve over baked potatoes with some chopped green onions or a sprinkle of herb mix. This can also be used as a salad dressing or dip.

GIO-KIO Fruit Dessert

Mix ¾ cup low-fat cottage cheese, 1 tablespoon honey, and ⅛ teaspoon ground nutmeg in a blender until smooth. Meanwhile, fill each individual serving dish with about ⅓ cup of cantaloupe cubes and ⅓ cup of honeydew melon cubes, mixed together. Top each dish with 1½ tablespoons of the cottage cheese mixture, and sprinkle each with a level teaspoon of wheat germ.

GIO-KIO Sandwich

Use whole-wheat, rye, or pumpernickel bread. Hold the mayo, but you may use 1 teaspoon of catsup or mustard, or 1 tablespoon of GIO-KIO French Dressing or Topping. Use no more than 2 ounces of lean meat such as beef, ham, or turkey. (Avoid all processed lunch meats.) Add no more than 1 ounce or slice of cheese. Add two or more of the following, heaped as high as you wish: lettuce, sliced tomato, sliced onion, dill pickles, bean sprouts, fresh mushrooms, spinach or other leafy greens. By varying these ingredients, you can produce an incredibly different array of sandwiches.

GIO-KIO Eggplant Supreme

Peel one small eggplant and slice it. Slice two small tomatoes into thick slices. Mix together ½ cup flour, 1 teaspoon salt, and ½ teaspoon oregano. Dip the vegetable slices into this mixture and fry them in a pan with one teaspoon of vegetable oil (preferably safflower). Fry till golden brown, then serve tomato slices on top of the eggplant slices. (Note: If you don't like eggplant, you can try zucchini, okra, or similar vegetable instead.)

GIO-KIO Pasta

Cook the noodles as usual, depending on the kind. You may use any size spaghetti, macaroni, or other pasta, preferably of the whole-wheat variety. After draining, mix with a little bit of the lowest-fat margarine you can find. Add per person 1 tablespoon of Parmesan or other grated cheese and a liberal sprinkle of garlic and onion powder. Mix all ingredients thoroughly in the pan while still warm. Serve immediately.

17

Fasting and Spiritual Growth

So far we have been looking at eating in positive and healthful ways, but there is another side of the story. There is also a time for fasting, for doing without food. As Ecclesiastes 3:1 says, "For everything there is a season, and a time for every matter under heaven."

Why Fast?

If food is good and meant to be enjoyed, why should we do without it at times?

Why do you think Jesus went into the wilderness and fasted for forty days and forty nights (Matthew 4:2)? Moses had a similar forty-day fast (Exodus 34:28) and so did Elijah (1 Kings 19:8). If they needed to fast that much before beginning major missions in life, do you think we might perhaps also need it to face some of our challenges?

Reasons for Fasting

To Humble Ourselves

Few things humble you like a fast (Psalms 35:13), particularly when combined with setting aside a special, uninterrupted time for prayer. When we are all wrapped up in the hustle and bustle of life, we often lose sight of deeper spiritual meanings. It's not so much that we consciously reject God and His Word, but we get so preoccupied that we may ignore Him.

When you fast and draw away from the world you strip a veil from before your eyes. You start to appreciate God's overall plan more and to understand your place in it. You discern that you are not the center of the universe, but that God is. You start to get a deeper insight into the spiritual ramifications of the events and concepts swirling around you. You realize more fully that you are not on earth to please yourself, have a good marriage and family, and grow rich. In short, your hunger reminds you that you are mortal and totally dependent on a loving God who can richly supply all your needs.

To Prepare for an Important Decision or Act

The followers of the church at Antioch were worshipping God and fasting and praying when the Holy Spirit told them to set aside Saul and Barnabas for their mission work (Acts 13:2–3). These two great missionaries then appointed elders to rule in each church, committing them to their new missions with prayer and fasting (Acts 14:23).

Fasting helps you concentrate in prayer. Have you ever noticed that in many prayer times your mind wanders to your own concerns, to the things you expect to do soon?

But when you have a special time of fasting, and you decide not to do anything else besides pray for those few hours (or days), you are better able to keep those other concerns out of your mind. You see the issues more clearly; you are more open to God's priorities and to His leading.

To Release Power

Do you remember the time when a little boy was possessed by a demon and the disciples could not cast it out? Jesus did so, and when they asked Him why they couldn't do it, He replied, "This kind does not go out except by prayer and fasting" (Matthew 17:21 NAS). Apparently, fasting helps strengthen the power and efficacy of prayer. Stubborn problems that won't yield to prayer alone may yet give way to prayer with fasting.

Present in all the aforementioned passages about fasting is the desire to have spiritual power descend on the person fasting and praying. For example, when the missionaries went out and the elders were appointed to church leadership, they needed more than just a good decision; they needed power to carry it out. Hence the fasting was combined with prayer.

To Lose Weight?

I *do not* recommend fasting to lose weight. True, you can lose weight fast that way, but you lose muscle as well as fat.[1] A normal low-calorie diet with some protein can help you lose more fat than a fasting situation in which you bring in no calories at all. Even though you burn more of your body's calorie store with a fast, more of it comes from protein (muscle). That's because you cannot break down fat and burn it without the presence of carbohydrate or protein. If you're not eating any of those two, your body rapidly burns up the tiny store of carbohydrate in your liver (called glycogen), and soon has to turn to the protein in your muscles. So, in a sense, fasting makes you "consume" your own muscle to burn fat and lose weight. It's better to protect your muscle and lose mostly fat.

Second, long-term fasting can completely throw off your vitamin and mineral balance. For this reason fasting *to lose weight* should be done only under the continuing guidance and supervision of a physician. In cases of serious obesity this is sometimes done. According to the *Guinness Book of World Records*, the record for fasting is held by Angus Barbieri of Scotland, who went over a year (382 days) without eating any solid food, though he did drink calorie-containing beverages and took vitamin supplements. He lost 294 pounds this way, declining from 472 to 178.

Third, I believe fasting is meant to be a spiritual regimen rather than a physical one. I think you should seek spiritual goals rather than earthly ones through a fast. Unless your doctor prescribes one, I think you would be missing the point of the experience if you looked at it simply as a quick weight-loss gimmick. As Isaiah 58:1–9 explains, a true fast that honors God must come from the heart, being drawn by pure motives to worship Him in this way.

How to Fast

Not Selfishly

As mentioned, the Isaiah passage explains that a fast should not be undertaken for wrong or selfish motives. As verse 4 says, "Fasting like yours this day will not make your voice to be heard on high." Jeremiah 14:12 expresses similar thoughts. Fasting and prayer give you a special time to commune with God. It is, however, a time for you to listen to His leading rather than to demand of Him what you want.

Not Openly

If you fast and pray openly, seeking the praise of men, that is the only reward you will get (Matthew 6:16–18). That approach honors self rather than God. Instead, fasting should be a private matter between you and the Lord. You should endeavor not to let others know of your sacrifice, "that your fasting may not be seen by men but by your Father who is in secret; and your Father who sees in secret will reward you" (v. 18).

Safely

I know some people who seem able to sustain a fast of several days or even a few weeks without ill effects. By about the third day of the fast, appetite is substantially suppressed. In other words, they don't even suffer much hunger, though they may feel weak and prefer to remain inactive.

But I know others who seem unable to skip even one meal without fairly dire consequences. They feel terribly hungry and deprived. They feel weak and unable to concentrate on anything. Such people often suffer from hypoglycemia, or low blood sugar. This means that they don't get enough energy to the brain, and their brain lets them know it by turning on all sorts of warning signals. For example, the heart races, perspiration increases, the muscles feel weak and shaky, and the person feels irritable, anxious, or dizzy. People experiencing such bad reactions should consider terminating their fast at once.

Furthermore, during a fast, you burn fat incompletely, producing an excess of ketones in the blood. This puts you into the state of ketosis, which can be uncomfortable and possibly even hazardous.

If you do decide to fast, I recommend that you skip just solid food. If you still drink nutritive fruit juices, they can supply the carbohydrate you need to burn fat more thoroughly and cleanly. Keep taking your regular vitamin and mineral pills, too. At the first sign of unusual disturbance—for example, an irregular heartbeat—get a small amount of food at once. If you experience any difficulties, see your physician.

Let me repeat, *I do not recommend fasting unless you are so advised by your physician.*

FASTING
CAN BRING YOU
CLOSER
TO GOD'S WILL

18

Getting Enough Spiritual Food

Anyone who is concerned only about physical food and bodily health is missing the most important part of life. Far more significant are spiritual food and health of the soul. There is not space to go into a complete theology but I do want to discuss a few topics that relate earthly food to heavenly "food," bodily health to spiritual health.

Only God Provides Life and Health

There are no magic pills or prescriptions for behavior and diet that can ensure continued earthly health and life. You could eat the best possible diet and take care of your exercise needs better than anyone else on the planet and still get hit by a truck, get shot, or fall prey to some new deadly disease.

As Proverbs 4:22 says, God's words "are life to him who finds them, and healing to all his flesh." If we seek God first, and His way for us to live (and eat) second, we might well live longer and healthier lives. But if we seek health first, and ignore God, there is no guarantee that any technique or approach will amount to anything.

Spiritual Bread Matters More Than Physical

We should get our priorities in order if we want to enjoy the best of both worlds. Seeking spiritual health first might help us find greater physical health as well. The other way around might make us lose out in both areas.

As Isaiah 55:2–3 says, "Why do you spend your money for that which is not bread. . . . Hearken diligently to me, and eat what is good. . . . Incline your ear, and come to me; hear, that your soul may live."

In John 6:51 Jesus says, "I am the living bread which came down from heaven; if any one eats of this bread, he will live for ever. . . ."

Our souls need bread, too. We should seek balanced spiritual meals more than physical ones. This means regular Bible study, prayer, communion with God, and thoughtful consideration of how we can apply God's principles in our daily lives.

Feed Others to Reduce Your Own Hunger

Our Bible tells us that we should be more concerned about feeding others than ourselves. Isaiah 58:7 says that part of the fast that honors God is "to share your bread with the hungry, and bring the homeless poor into your house. . . ." Ezekiel 18:7 says that the righteous person "gives his bread to the hungry and covers the naked with a garment." And James 2:15–16 says that if we see people who are hungry and have other needs, we shouldn't just wish them well but do something to help them out in a tangible way.

What all these verses are saying is that the person who belongs to God shouldn't just look after himself and his own wants. He should be sensitive to the needs of others and reach out to help them in a sharing way.

Let's face it: Even though the GIO-KIO plan lets you eat all you want of the right items and anything you want as long as you restrict the amounts, it doesn't let you eat all you want of everything you want. That would be no diet at all, but simply binge eating. Therefore, no matter how great you feel on this

plan and how much you love seeing that fat slip away, there
will be times when you will feel dissatisfied about what you are
giving up. That extra slice of strawberry cheesecake will sing
out to you.

What better way to forget about minor hunger and deprivation than to seek out and help those who suffer with serious
unmet needs? If you haven't already, why don't you consider
doing more to help the hungry in your community and around
the world? Your local church, denominational ministry, and
various nondenominational and secular groups have many
ways you can contribute your money, time, and ideas.

Earn Blessings by Feeding Others

As Proverbs 22:9 puts it, "He who has a bountiful eye will be
blessed, for he shares his bread with the poor." Ecclesiastes
11:1 says, "Cast your bread upon the waters, for you will find it
after many days." And in Acts 20:35 Jesus says, "It is more
blessed to give than to receive."

When we help others, we are not simply sacrificing ourselves
according to some ritual. We are actually earning blessings for
ourselves at the same time! Of course, to give to others with the
sole motive of expecting something in return is to miss the
point completely.

If we respond in love and compassion to the needs of others
according to God's will, as unselfishly as we can, we will yet
reap wonderful rewards and blessings in return.

The Fruit of Eternal Life

The most wonderful food of all—the fruit of eternal life—
cannot be earned. God offers it to us as a free gift, and we must
either accept it on His terms or reject it.

Revelation 2:7 states that only God can "grant to eat from the
tree of life, which is in the paradise of God." Revelation 22:2
describes the tree of life further as a great tree in heaven
yielding twelve crops of fruit and leaves "for the healing of the
nations."

Have you accepted God's free gifts?

As Jesus says in Revelation 3:20, "Behold, I stand at the door and knock; if any one hears my voice and opens the door, I will come in to him and eat with him, and he with me." Jesus will not force the door open, but He will enter as soon as you open and let Him.

FEED OTHERS
AND
REDUCE
YOUR OWN HUNGER

Source Notes

Chapter 1   **Rich Food, Poor Body**

1. H. W. F. Saggs, *The Greatness That Was Babylon* (New York: Hawthorn, 1962), pp. 172–76.

2. F. M. Sacks, B. Rosner, and E. H. Kass, "Blood Pressure in Vegetarians," *American Journal of Epidemiology*, 100 (1974): 390–98.

3. I. L. Rouse, L. J. Beilin, B. K. Armstrong, and R. Vandongen, "Blood Pressure Lowering Effect of a Vegetarian Diet: A Controlled Trial in Normotensive Subjects," *Lancet* 1 (1983): 5–10.

4. F. M. Sacks, A. Donner, W. P. Castelli, J. Gronemeyer, P. Pietka, H. S. Margolius, L. Landsberg, and E. H. Kass, "Effect of Ingestion of Meat on Plasma Cholesterol of Vegetarians," *Journal of the American Medical Association*, 246 (1981): 640–44.

5. B. N. Ames, "Dietary Carcinogens and Anticarcinogens," *Science*, 221 (1983): 1256–64.

6. *World Almanac and Book of Facts* (New York: Newspaper Enterprise Association, 1986), p. 780.

7. Adapted from W. P. Castelli, "Epidemiology of Coronary Heart Disease: The Framingham Study," *American Journal of Medicine*, vol. 76 (2A) (1984): 4–12.

8. S. M. Berger, "How to Lose Weight Safely," *Parade*, 10 November 1985, pp. 12–13.

9. National Institutes of Health, *Health Implications of Obesity* (Bethesda, Maryland: Consensus Development Conference Statement, vol. 5, no. 9, 1985).

10. R. A. Arky, "The Role of Diet and Exercise in the Care of Patients with Diabetes Mellitus," in *Genetic Environmental Interaction in Diabetes Mellitus*, ed. J. S. Melish, J. Hanna, and S. Baba (Amsterdam: Excerpta Medica, 1982).

Chapter 2   **Do You Need to Lose Weight?**

1. W. H. Dietz and S. L. Gortmaker, "Do We Fatten Our Children at the Television Set? Obesity and Television Viewing in Children and Adolescents," *Pediatrics*, 75 (1985): 807–12.

2. L. Page and L. J. Fincher, *Food and Your Weight*, Home and Garden Bulletin no. 74 (Washington, D.C.: U.S. Government Printing Office, 1967), p. 2.

Chapter 4   **The Purpose of Food**

1. M. E. Lowenberg, E. N. Todhunter, E. D. Wilson, J. R. Savage, and J. L. Lubawski, *Food and Man*, 2nd ed. (New York: Wiley, 1974), p. 35.

2. *Ibid.*, p. 45.

Chapter 5   What Is a Good Diet?

1. P. Felig, "Very-Low-Calorie Protein Diets," *New England Journal of Medicine,* 310 (1984): 589–91.

2. *Ibid.,* 590.

3. F. S. Bodenheimer, *Insects as Human Food* (The Hague: Dr. W. Junk, 1951).

Chapter 6   Avoid Excess Fat

1. E. M. N. Hamilton, E. N. Whitney, and F. S. Sizer, *Nutrition: Concepts and Controversies,* 3rd ed. (New York: West, 1982), p. 104.

2. D. I. Gregorio, L. J. Emrich, S. Graham, J. R. Marshall, and T. Nemoto, "Dietary Fat Consumption and Survival among Women with Breast Cancer," *Journal of the National Cancer Institute,* 75 (1985): 37–41.

Chapter 7   Avoid Excess Sugar

1. S. O. Welsh and R. M. Marston, "Review of Trends in Food Use in the United States, 1909 to 1980," *Journal of the American Dietetic Association* 81 (1982): 120–25.

2. W. M. Pardridge, "Potential Effects of the Dipeptide Sweetener Aspartame on the Brain," in *Nutrition and the Brain,* vol. 7, ed. R. J. Wurtman and J. J. Wurtman (New York: Raven Press, 1986), pp. 199–241.

3. A. Lindesmith, "Psychology of Addiction," in *Principles of Psychopharmacology,* ed. W. G. Clark and J. D. Giudice (New York: Academic Press, 1970) pp. 471–76.

Chapter 8   Avoid Excess Protein

1. B. M. Brenner, T. W. Meyer, and T. H. Hostetter, "Dietary Protein Intake and the Progressive Nature of Kidney Disease," *New England Journal of Medicine,* 307 (1982): 652–59.

2. P. Felig, "Very-Low-Calorie Protein Diets," *New England Journal of Medicine,* 310 (1984): 589–91.

3. Hamilton, Whitney, and Sizer, *Nutrition: Concepts and Controversies,* p. 141.

4. "Immunological Studies of Fish Oil," *Harvard Medical Area Focus,* 26 September 1985, pp. 1–6.

Chapter 9   Avoid Excess Salt

1. Hamilton, Whitney, and Sizer, *Nutrition: Concepts and Controversies,* p. 284.

Chapter 10   The Need for Carbohydrates

1. Hamilton, Whitney, and Sizer, *Nutrition: Concepts and Controversies,* p. 69.

2. *Ibid.* p. 70.

3. J. Himms-Hagen, "Determinants of Human Obesity," *Clinical Nutrition,* 1(1) (1982): 4–8.

Chapter 11   The Need for Water

1. H. T. Randall, "Water, Electrolytes and Acid-Base Balance," in *Modern Nutrition in Health and Disease,* ed. R. S. Goodhart and M. E. Shils, 6th ed. (Philadelphia: Lea & Febiger, 1980), p. 356.

2. *Ibid.,* p. 360.

3. A. H. Ensminger, M. E. Ensminger, J. E. Konlande, and J. R. K. Robson, *Foods & Nutrition Encyclopedia* (Clovis, California: Pegus, 1983), p. 2285.

4. *Encyclopedia of Sport Sciences and Medicine* (New York: Macmillan, 1971), pp. 129–30.

5. American Dietetic Association, "Nutrition and Physical Fitness," in *Sourcebook on Food and Nutrition,* 3rd ed. (Chicago: Marquis Academic Media, 1982), p. 253.

6. M. E. Shils and H. T. Randall, "Diet and Nutrition in the Care of the Surgical Patient," in *Modern Nutrition in Health and Disease,* 6th ed., ed. R. S. Goodhart and M. E. Shils (Philadelphia: Lea & Febiger, 1980), p. 1106.

7. F. J. Stare and M. McWilliams, *Living Nutrition* (New York: Wiley, 1973), p. 303.

8. *Encyclopedia of Sport Sciences and Medicine* (New York: Macmillan, 1971), p. 130.

9. *Ibid.*

10. *Ibid.*

11. V. M. Sharma, K. Sridharan, G. Pichan, and M. R. Panwar, "Influence of Heat-Stress Induced Dehydration on Mental Functions," *Ergonomics,* 29 (1986): 791–99.

12. *Encyclopedia of Sport Sciences and Medicine* (New York: Macmillan, 1971), p. 131.

13. A. D. Claremont, D. L. Costill, W. Fink, and P. Van Handel, "Heat Tolerance Following Diuretic Induced Dehydration," *Medicine and Science in Sports,* 8 (1976): 239–43.

14. "The Nutritional Origin of Cataracts," *Nutrition Reviews,* 42 (1984): 377–79.

15. Shils and Randall, *Modern Nutrition,* p. 1105.

16. *Ibid.*

17. *Ibid.,* p. 1110.

Chapter 12   Breaking the Tyranny of Gluttony

1. H. Lehnert, D. K. Reinstein, B. W. Strowbridge, and R. J. Wurtman, "Neurochemical and Behavioral Consequences of Acute, Uncontrollable Stress: Effects of Dietary Tyrosine," *Brain Research,* 303 (1984): 215–23.

2. B. Spring, O. Maller, J. Wurtman, L. Digman, and L. Cozolino, "Effects of Protein and Carbohydrate Meals on Mood and Performance: Interactions with Sex and Age," *Journal of Psychiatric Research*, 17 (1983): 155–67.

3. R. J. Wurtman and J. J. Wurtman, "Carbohydrate Craving, Obesity and Brain Serotonin," *Appetite*, 7 (1986): 99–103.

4. Spring et al. "Effects of Protein," pp. 155–67.

Chapter 13   The Fun Way to Lose Weight

1. R. S. Paffenbarger, R. T. Hyde, A. L. Wing, and C. Hsieh, "Physical Activity, All-Cause Mortality, and Longevity of College Alumni," *New England Journal of Medicine*, 314 (1986): 605–13.

2. N. R. Carlson, *Physiology of Behavior*, 2nd ed. (Boston: Allyn and Bacon, 1981).

3. A. H. Ismail and L. E. Trachtman, "Jogging the Imagination," *Psychology Today*, March 1973, pp. 78–82.

4. M. Elsayed, A. H. Ismail, and R. J. Young, "Intellectual Differences of Adult Men Related to Age and Physical Fitness Before and After an Exercise Program," *Journal of Gerontology*, 35 (1980): 383–87.

Chapter 14   Diet, Health, and Sex

1. R. Virag, "International Society for Impotence Research in Paris," *Parade*, 19 August 1984, p. 16.

2. F. Field, "How Many Calories in a Kiss?" *Reader's Digest*, December 1985, 181–82.

3. A. Keys, J. Brozek, A. Henschel, O. Mickelson, and H. L. Taylor, *The Biology of Human Starvation* (Minneapolis: University of Minnesota Press, 1950).

Chapter 15   Changing Food Habits

1. T. R. Lankford and P. M. Jacobs-Steward, *Foundations of Normal and Therapeutic Nutrition* (New York: Wiley, 1986).

2. *Ibid.*

3. E. Rubin and H. Rottenberg, "Ethanol-Induced Injury and Adaptation in Biological Membranes," *Federation Proceedings*, 41 (1982): 2465–471.

4. "Caffeine," *Food Technology*, 37 (1983): 87–91.

5. *Ibid.*

6. *Ibid.*

7. P. W. Curatolo and D. Robertson, "The Health Consequences of Caffeine," *Annals of Internal Medicine*, 98 (Part 1) (1983): 641–53.

8. Ames, "Dietary Carcinogens," p. 1259.

Chapter 17   Fasting and Spiritual Growth

1. Hamilton, Whitney, and Sizer, *Nutrition: Concepts and Controversies*, pp. 166–67.

Appendix A

Calorie Counts for Various Foods

Remember: You Can Eat *Anything* You Want on This Diet

As a rule, *you do not count calories on this diet and health plan.* You only need to count calories for your daily dessert treat to ensure that you do not exceed 200 calories per treat.

These tables have a second purpose. As you go beyond the period of Daniel's ten-day diet challenge in chapter 16, you will need to find substitute foods that you like so you can put more variety into your diet. These tables will help you recognize the lower-calorie alternatives among the various food groups. But *don't* waste time actually totaling up calories. Instead, listen to your body and the instinctive hunger/satiation system that God built in. If you eat the right foods consistently, it will not steer you wrong.

These tables are reprinted from *Food and Your Weight* (Washington, D.C.: U.S. Department of Agriculture: Home and Garden Bulletin no. 274, 1967), pp. 17–30.

Milk, Cheese, and Ice Cream

		Number of calories
Fluid milk:		
Whole	1 cup or glass	160
Skim (fresh or nonfat dry reconstituted)	1 cup or glass	90
Buttermilk	1 cup or glass	90
Evaporated (undiluted)	½ cup	170
Condensed, sweetened (undiluted)	½ cup	490
Half-and-half (milk and cream)	1 cup	325
	1 tablespoon	20
Cream, light	1 tablespoon	30
Cream, heavy whipping	1 tablespoon	55
Yogurt (made from partially skimmed milk)	1 cup	120

Cheese:

American,	1 ounce	115
Cheddar-type	1-inch cube (⅗ ounce)	70
	½ cup, grated (2 ounces)	225
Process American, Cheddar-type	1 ounce	105
Blue-mold (or Roquefort-type)	1 ounce	105
Cottage, not creamed	2 tablespoons (1 ounce)	25
Cottage, creamed	2 tablespoons (1 ounce)	30
Cream	2 tablespoons (1 ounce)	105
Parmesan, dry, grated	2 tablespoons (⅓ ounce)	40
Swiss	1 ounce	105

Milk beverages:

Cocoa (all milk)	1 cup	235
Chocolate-flavored milk drink	1 cup	190
Malted milk	1 cup	280
Chocolate milk shake	One 12-ounce container	520
Ice cream, plain	1 container (3½ fluid ounces)	130
Ice milk	½ cup (4 fluid ounces)	140
Ice cream soda, chocolate	1 large glass	455

Meat, Poultry, Fish, Eggs Dry Beans and Peas, Nuts

		Number of Calories
Meat, cooked, without bone:		
Beef:		
Pot roast or braised:		
Lean and fat	3 ounces (1 thick or 2 thin slices, 4 by 2½ inches)	245
Lean only	2½ ounces (1 thick or 2 thin slices, 4 by 2 inches)	140
Oven roast:		
Cut having relatively large proportion of fat to lean:		
Lean and fat	3 ounces (1 thick or 2 thin slices, 4 by 2½ inches)	375
Lean only	2 ounces (1 thick or 2 thin slices, 4 by 1½ inches)	140

Cut having relatively low proportion of fat to lean:		
Lean and fat	3 ounces (1 thick or 2 thin slices, 4 by 2½ inches)	165
Lean only	2½ ounces (1 thick or 2 thin slices, 4 by 2 inches)	115
Steak, broiled:		
Lean and fat	3 ounces (1 piece, 4 by 2½ inches by ½ inch)	330
Lean only	2 ounces (1 piece, 4 by 1½ inches by ½ inch)	115
Hamburger patty:		
Regular ground beef	3-ounce patty (about 4 patties per pound of raw meat)	245
Lean ground round	3-ounce patty (about 4 patties per pound of raw meat)	185
Corned beef, canned	3 ounces (1 piece, 4 by 2½ inches by ½ inch)	185
Corned beef hash, canned	3 ounces (scant half cup)	155
Dried beef, chipped	2 ounces (about ⅓ cup)	115
Meat loaf	2 ounces (1 piece, 4 by 2½ inches by ½ inch)	115
Beef and vegetable stew	½ cup	105
Beef potpie, baked	1 pie, 4¼ inch diameter, about 8 ounces before baking	560
Chile con carne, canned:		
Without beans	½ cup	255
With beans	½ cup	170
Veal:		
Cutlet, broiled, meat only	3 ounces (1 piece, 4 by 2½ inches by ½ inch)	185
Lamb:		
Chop (about 2½ chops to a pound, as purchased):		
Lean and fat	4 ounces	400
Lean only	2⅗ ounces	140
Roast, leg:		
Lean and fat	3 ounces (1 thick or 2 thin slices, 3½ by 3 inches)	235

Lean only	2½ ounces (1 thick or 2 thin slices, 3½ by 2½ inches)	130
Pork:		
Fresh:		
Chop (about 3 chops to a pound, as purchased):		
Lean and fat	2⅓ ounces	260
Lean only	2 ounces	155
Roast, loin:		
Lean and fat	3 ounces (1 thick or 2 thin slices, 4 by 2½ inches)	310
Lean only	2⅖ ounces (1 thick or 2 thin slices, 3 by 2½ inches)	175
Cured Ham:		
Lean and fat	3 ounces (1 thick or 2 thin slices, 4 by 2 inches)	245
Lean only	2⅕ ounces (1 thick or 2 thin slices, 3½ by 2 inches)	120
Bacon, broiled or fried	2 very thin slices	100
Sausage and variety and luncheon meats:		
Bologna sausage	2 ounces (2 very thin slices, 4 inches in diameter)	170
Liver sausage (liverwurst)	2 ounces (4 very thin slices, 3 inches in diameter)	175
Vienna sausage, canned	2 ounces (4 to 5 sausages)	135
Pork sausage, bulk	2 ounces (1 patty, 2 inches in diameter), (4 to 5 patties per pound, raw)	270
Liver, beef, fried (includes fat for frying)	2 ounces (1 thick piece, 3 by 2½ inches)	130
Heart, beef, braised, trimmed of fat	3 ounces (1 thick piece, 4 by 2½ inches)	160
Tongue, beef, braised	3 ounces (1 thick slice, 4 by 2½ inches)	210
Frankfurter	1 frankfurter	155
Boiled ham (luncheon meat)	2 ounces (2 very thin slices, 3½ by 3½ inches)	135

Spiced ham, canned	2 ounces (2 thin slices, 3 by 2½ inches)	165
Poultry, cooked, without bone:		
Chicken:		
Broiled	3 ounces (about ¼ of a small broiler	185
Fried	½ breast, 2⅘ ounces	155
	1 leg (thigh and drumstick), 3 ounces	225
Canned	3½ ounces (½ cup)	200
Poultry pie (with potatoes, peas, and gravy)	1 small pie, 4¼ inches in diameter (about 8 ounces before cooking)	535
Fish and shellfish:		
Bluefish, baked	3 ounces (1 piece, 3½ by 2 inches by ½ inch)	135
Clams, shelled:		
Raw, meat only	3 ounces (about 4 medium clams)	65
Canned, clams and juice	3 ounces (1 scant half cup, 3 medium clams and juice)	45
Crab meat, canned or cooked	3 ounces, ½ cup	85
Fish sticks, breaded, cooked, frozen (including breading and fat for frying)	4 ounces (5 fish sticks)	200
Haddock, fried (including fat for frying)	3 ounces (1 fillet, 4 by 2½ inches by ½ inch)	140
Mackerel:		
Broiled	3 ounces (1 piece, 4 by 3 inches by ½ inch)	200
Canned	3 ounces, solids and liquid (about ⅗ cup)	155
Ocean perch, fried (including egg, breadcrumbs, and fat for frying)	3 ounces (1 piece, 4 by 2½ inches by ½ inch)	195
Oysters, shucked:		
Raw, meat only	½ cup (6 to 10 medium-size oysters, selects)	80
Salmon:		
Broiled or baked	4 ounces (1 steak, 4½ by 2½ inches by ½ inch)	205
Canned (pink)	3 ounces, solids and liquid, about ⅗ cup	120

Sardines, canned in oil	3 ounces, drained solids (5 to 7 medium sardines)	175
Shrimp, canned, meat only	3 ounces (about 17 medium shrimp)	100
Tuna fish, canned in oil, meat only	3 ounces (about ⅖ cup)	170
Eggs:		
Fried (including fat for frying)	1 large egg	100
Hard or soft cooked, boiled	1 large egg	80
Scrambled or omelet (including milk and fat for cooking)	1 large egg	110
Poached	1 large egg	80
Dry beans and peas:		
Red kidney beans, canned or cooked	½ cup, solids and liquid	115
Lima, cooked	½ cup, solids and liquid	130
Baked beans, with tomato or molasses:		
With pork	½ cup	160
Without pork	½ cup	155
Nuts:		
Almonds, shelled	2 tablespoons (about 13 to 15 almonds)	105
Brazil nuts, shelled, broken pieces	2 tablespoons	115
Cashew nuts, roasted	2 tablespoons (about 4 to 5 nuts)	95
Coconut:		
Fresh, shredded meat	2 tablespoons	40
Dried, shredded, sweetened	2 tablespoons	45
Peanuts, roasted, shelled	2 tablespoons	105
Peanut butter	1 tablespoon	95
Pecans, shelled halves	2 tablespoons (about 12 to 14 halves)	95
Walnuts, shelled:		
Black or native, chopped	2 tablespoons	100
English or Persian, halves	2 tablespoons (about 7 to 12 halves)	80

Vegetables and Fruits

		Number of calories
Vegetables:		
Asparagus, cooked or canned	6 medium spears or ½ cup cut spears	20
Beans:		
Lima, green, cooked or canned	½ cup	80
Snap, green, wax or yellow, cooked or canned	½ cup	15
Beets, cooked or canned	½ cup, diced	30
Beet greens, cooked	½ cup	15
Broccoli, cooked	½ cup flower stalks	20
Brussels sprouts, cooked	½ cup	20
Cabbage:		
Raw	½ cup, shredded	10
	1 wedge, 3½ by 4½ inches	25
Coleslaw (with mayonnaise-type salad dressing)	½ cup	60
Cooked	½ cup	20
Carrots:		
Raw	1 carrot, 5½ inches by 1 inch in diameter, or 25 thin slices	20
	½ cup, grated	20
Cooked	½ cup, diced	20
Cauliflower, cooked	½ cup flower buds	10
Celery, raw	2 large stalks, 8 inches long, or 3 small stalks, 5 inches long	10
Chard, cooked	½ cup	15
Collards, cooked	½ cup	30
Corn:		
On cob, cooked	1 ear, 5 inches long	70
Kernels, cooked or canned	½ cup	85
Cress, garden, cooked	½ cup	20
Cucumbers, raw, pared	6 slices, ⅛ inch thick, center section	5
Kale, cooked	½ cup	15
Kohlrabi, cooked	½ cup	20
Lettuce, raw	2 large or 4 small leaves	10
Mushrooms, canned	½ cup	20
Mustard greens, cooked	½ cup	20

Okra, cooked	4 pods, 3 inches long, ⅝ inch in diameter	10
Onions:		
Young, green, raw	6 small, without tops	20
Mature:	1 onion, 2½ inches in	40
Raw	diameter	
	1 tablespoon, chopped	5
Cooked	½ cup	30
Parsnips, cooked	½ cup	50
Peas, green:		
Cooked or canned	½ cup	60
Peppers, green:		
Raw or cooked	1 medium	10
Potatoes:		
Baked	1 medium, 2½ inches in diameter (5 ounces raw)	90
Boiled	½ cup, diced	50
Chips (including fat for frying)	10 medium, 2 inches in diameter	115
French-fried (including fat for frying):		
Ready-to-eat	10 pieces, 2 inches by ½ inch by ½ inch	155
Frozen, heated, ready-to-serve	10 pieces, 2 inches by ½ inch by ½ inch	125
Hashbrowned	½ cup	225
Mashed:		
Milk added	½ cup	60
Milk and fat added	½ cup	90
Pan-fried, beginning with raw potatoes	½ cup	230
Radishes, raw	4 small	5
Sauerkraut, canned	½ cup	20
Spinach, cooked or canned	½ cup	20
Squash:		
Summer, cooked	½ cup	15
Winter, baked, mashed	½ cup	65
Sweet potatoes:		
Baked in jacket	1 medium, 5 by 2 inches (6 ounces raw)	155
Canned, vacuum or solid pack	½ cup	120
Tomatoes:		
Raw	1 medium, 2 by 2½ inches (about ⅓ pound)	35
Cooked or canned	½ cup	25

Tomato juice, canned	½ cup	20
Turnips, cooked	½ cup	20
Turnip greens, cooked	½ cup	15
Fruits:		
Apples, raw	1 medium, 2½ inches in diameter (about ⅓ pound)	70
Apple juice, canned	½ cup	60
Applesauce:		
Sweetened	½ cup	115
Unsweetened	½ cup	50
Apricots:		
Raw	3 (about 12 to a pound, as purchased)	55
Canned:		
Water pack	½ cup, halves and liquid	45
Heavy syrup pack	½ cup, halves and syrup	110
Dried, cooked, un-sweetened	½ cup, fruit and juice	120
Frozen, sweetened	½ cup	125
Avocados:		
California varieties:	½ of a 10-ounce avocado (3⅓ by 4¼ inches)	185
Florida varieties	½ of a 13-ounce avocado (4 by 3 inches)	160
Bananas, raw	1 banana (6 by 1½ inches, about ⅓ pound)	85
Berries:		
Blackberries, raw	½ cup	40
Blueberries, raw	½ cup	40
Raspberries:		
Fresh, red, raw	½ cup	35
Frozen, red, sweetened	½ cup	120
Fresh, black, raw	½ cup	50
Strawberries:		
Fresh, raw	½ cup	30
Frozen, sweetened	½ cup, sliced	140
Cantaloupe, raw	½ melon, 5 inches in diameter	60
Cherries:		
Raw:		
Sour	½ cup	30
Sweet	½ cup	40
Cranberry sauce, canned, sweetened	1 tablespoon	25
Cranberry juice cocktail, canned	½ cup	80

Dates, "fresh" and dried, pitted, cut	½ cup	245
Figs:		
Raw	3 small (1½ inches in diameter, about ¼ pound)	90
Canned, heavy syrup	½ cup	110
Dried	1 large (2 inches by 1 inch)	60
Fruit cocktail, canned in heavy syrup	½ cup	100
Grapefruit:		
Raw:		
White	½ medium (4¼ inches in diameter, no. 64s)	55
	½ cup sections	40
Pink or red	½ medium (4¼ inches in diameter, no. 64s)	60
Canned:		
Water pack	½ cup	35
Syrup pack	½ cup	90
Grapefruit juice:		
Raw	½ cup	50
Canned:		
Unsweetened	½ cup	50
Sweetened	½ cup	65
Frozen concentrate, diluted, ready-to-serve:		
Unsweetened	½ cup	50
Sweetened	½ cup	60
Grapes, raw:		
American type (including Concord, Delaware, Niagara, and Scuppernong), slip skin	1 bunch (3½ by 3 inches; about 3½ ounces) ½ cup, with skins and seeds	45 30
European type (including Malaga, Muscat, Thompson seedless, and Flame Tokay), adherent skin	½ cup	50
Grape juice, bottled	½ cup	80
Honeydew melon, raw	1 wedge, 2 by 7 inches	50

Lemon juice, raw or canned	½ cup	30
	1 tablespoon	5
Lemonade, frozen concentrate, sweetened, diluted, ready-to-serve	½ cup	55
Oranges, raw	1 orange, 3 inches in diameter	75
Orange juice:		
Raw	½ cup	55
Canned, unsweetened	½ cup	60
Frozen concentrate, diluted, ready-to-serve	½ cup	55
Peaches:		
Raw	1 medium, 2 inches in diameter (about ¼ pound)	35
	½ cup, sliced	30
Canned:		
Water pack	½ cup	40
Heavy syrup pack	½ cup	100
Dried, cooked, un-sweetened	½ cup (5 to 6 halves and 3 tablespoons syrup)	110
Frozen, sweetened	½ cup	105
Pears:		
Raw	1 pear, 3 by 2½ inches in diameter	100
Canned in heavy syrup	½ cup	100
Pineapple:		
Raw	½ cup, diced	40
Canned in heavy syrup:		
Crushed	½ cup	100
Sliced	2 small or 1 large slice and 2 tablespoons juice	90
Pineapple juice, canned	½ cup	70
Plums:		
Raw	1 plum, 2 inches in diameter (about 2 ounces)	25
Canned, syrup pack	½ cup	100
Prunes, dried, cooked:		
Unsweetened	½ cup (8 to 9 prunes and 2 tablespoons liquid)	150

Sweetened	½ cup (8 to 9 prunes and 2 tablespoons liquid)	255
Prune juice, canned	½ cup	100
Raisins, dried	½ cup	230
Rhubarb, cooked, sweetened	½ cup	190
Tangerine, raw	1 medium, 2½ inches in diameter (about ¼ pound)	40
Tangerine juice, canned	½ cup	50
Watermelon, raw	1 wedge, 4 by 8 inches long (about 2 pounds, including rind)	115

Bread and Cereals

		Number of calories
Bread:		
Cracked wheat	1 slice, ½ inch thick	60
Raisin	1 slice, ½ inch thick	60
Rye	1 slice, ½ inch thick	55
White	1 slice, ½ inch thick	60
Whole-wheat	1 slice, ½ inch thick	55
Other baked goods:		
Baking powder biscuit	1 biscuit, 2½ inches in diameter	140
Crackers:		
Graham	4 small or 2 medium	55
Saltines	2 crackers, 2 inches square	35
Soda	2 crackers, 2½ inches square	50
Oyster	10 crackers	45
Doughnuts (cake type)	1 doughnut	125
Muffins:		
Plain	1 muffin, 2¾ inches in diameter	140
Bran	1 muffin, 2¾ inches in diameter	130
Corn	1 muffin, 2¾ inches in diameter	150
Pancakes (griddle cakes):		
Wheat (home recipe)	1 cake, 4 inches in diameter	60
Buckwheat (with buckwheat pancake mix)	1 cake, 4 inches in diameter	55

Pizza (cheese)	5½-inch sector, ⅛ of a 14-inch pie	185
Pretzels	5 small sticks	20
Rolls:		
Plain, pan	1 roll (16 ounces per dozen)	115
Hard, round	1 roll (22 ounces per dozen)	160
Sweet, pan	1 roll (18 ounces per dozen)	135
Rye wafers	2 wafers, 1⅞ by 3½ inches	45
Waffles	1 waffle, 4½ by 5½ by ½ inch	210
Cakes, cookies, pies (See Desserts)		
Cereals and other grain products:		
Bran flakes (40 percent bran)	1 ounce (about ⅘ cup)	85
Corn, puffed, pre-sweetened	1 ounce (about 1 cup)	110
Corn, shredded	1 ounce (about ⅘ cup)	110
Corn flakes	1 ounce (about 1⅓ cups)	110
Corn grits, degermed, cooked	¾ cup	90
Farina, cooked	¾ cup	75
Macaroni, cooked	¾ cup	115
Macaroni and cheese	½ cup	235
Noodles, cooked	¾ cup	150
Oat cereal (mixture mainly oat flour)	1 ounce (about 1⅛ cups)	115
Oatmeal or rolled oats, cooked	¾ cup	100
Rice, cooked	¾ cup	140
Rice flakes	1 cup (about 1 ounce)	115
Rice, puffed	1 cup (about ½ ounce)	55
Spaghetti, cooked	¾ cup	115
Spaghetti with meatballs	¾ cup	250
Spaghetti in tomato sauce, with cheese	¾ cup	195
Wheat, puffed	1 ounce (about 2⅛ cups)	105
Wheat, puffed, pre-sweetened	1 ounce (about 2⅛ cups)	105
Wheat, rolled, cooked	¾ cup	130
Wheat, shredded, plain (long, round, or bite-size)	1 ounce (1 large biscuit or about ½ cup bite-size)	100

Wheat flakes	1 ounce (about ¾ cup)	100
Wheat flours:		
Whole-wheat	¾ cup, stirred	300
All-purpose (or family) flour	¾ cup, sifted	300
Wheat germ	¾ cup, stirred	185

Fats, Oils, and Related Products

		Number of calories
Butter or margarine	1 tablespoon	100
	1 pat or square (64 per pound)	50
Cooking fats:		
Vegetable	1 tablespoon	110
Lard	1 tablespoon	125
Salad or cooking oils	1 tablespoon	125
Salad dressings:		
French	1 tablespoon	60
Blue cheese, French	1 tablespoon	80
Home-cooked, boiled	1 tablespoon	30
Low-calorie	1 tablespoon	15
Mayonnaise	1 tablespoon	110
Salad dressing, commercial, plain (mayonnaise-type)	1 tablespoon	65
Thousand Island	1 tablespoon	75

Sugars, Sweets, and Related Products

		Number of calories
Candy:		
Caramels	1 ounce (3 medium caramels)	115
Chocolate creams	1 ounce (2 to 3 pieces, 35 to a pound)	125
Chocolate, milk, sweetened	1-ounce bar	150
Chocolate, milk, sweetened, with almonds	1-ounce bar	150
Chocolate mints	1 ounce (1 to 2 mints, 20 to a pound)	115
Fudge, milk chocolate, plain	1 ounce (1 piece, 1 to 1½ inches square)	115
Gumdrops	1 ounce (about 2½ large or 20 small)	100

Hard candy	1 ounce (3 to 4 candy balls, ¾ inch in diameter)	110
Jelly beans	1 ounce (10 beans)	105
Marshmallows	1 ounce (3 to 4 marshmallows, 60 to a pound)	90
Peanut brittle	1 ounce (1½ pieces, 2½ by 1¼ inches by ⅜ inch)	120
Syrup, honey, molasses:		
Chocolate syrup	1 tablespoon	50
Honey, strained or extracted	1 tablespoon	65
Molasses, cane, light	1 tablespoon	50
Syrup, table blends	1 tablespoon	60
Jelly	1 tablespoon	55
Jam, marmalade, preserves	1 tablespoon	55
Sugar: white, granulated, or brown	1 teaspoon	15

Soups

		Number of calories
Bean with pork	1 cup	170
Beef noodle	1 cup	70
Bouillon, broth, and consommé	1 cup	30
Chicken noodle	1 cup	65
Clam chowder	1 cup	85
Cream of asparagus	1 cup	155
Cream of mushroom	1 cup	135
Minestrone	1 cup	105
Oyster stew	1 cup (3 or 4 oysters)	200
Tomato	1 cup	90
Vegetable with beef broth	1 cup	80

Desserts

		Number of calories
Apple betty	½ cup	170
Cakes:		
Angel food	2-inch sector (1/12 of 8-inch round cake)	110

Butter cakes:		
Plain, without icing	1 piece, 3 by 2 by 1½ inches	200
	1 cupcake, 2¾ inches in diameter	145
Plain, with chocolate icing	2-inch sector (1/16 of 10-inch round layer cake)	370
	1 cupcake, 2¾ inches in diameter	185
Chocolate, with chocolate icing	2-inch sector (1/16 of 10-inch round layer cake)	445
Fruitcake, dark	1 piece, 2 by 2 inches by ½ inch	115
Gingerbread	1 piece, 2 by 2 by 2 inches	175
Pound cake	1 slice, 2¾ by 3 inches by 5/8 inch	140
Sponge cake	2-inch sector (1/12 of 8-inch round cake)	120
Cookies, plain and assorted	1 cookie, 3 inches in diameter	120
Cornstarch pudding	½ cup	140
Custard, baked	½ cup	140
Fig bars, small	1 fig bar	55
Fruit ice	½ cup	75
Gelatin dessert, plain, ready-to-serve	½ cup	70
Ice cream, plain	1 container (3½ fluid ounces)	130
Ice milk	½ cup (4 fluid ounces)	140
Pies:		
Apple	4-inch sector (1/7 of 9-inch pie)	345
Cherry	4-inch sector (1/7 of 9-inch pie)	355
Custard	4-inch sector (1/7 of 9-inch pie)	280
Lemon meringue	4-inch sector (1/7 of 9-inch pie)	305
Mince	4-inch sector (1/7 of 9-inch pie)	365
Pumpkin	4-inch sector (1/7 of 9-inch pie)	275
Prune whip	½ cup	105
Rennet dessert pudding, ready-to-serve	½ cup	130
Sherbet	½ cup	130

Beverages (not including milk beverages and fruit juices)

		Number of calories
Carbonated Beverages:		
Ginger ale	8-ounce glass	70

Cola-type	8-ounce glass	95
Alcoholic beverages:		
Beer, 3.6 percent alcohol by weight	8-ounce glass	100
Whisky, gin, rum:		
100-proof	1 jigger (1½ ounces)	125
90-proof	1 jigger (1½ ounces)	110
86-proof	1 jigger (1½ ounces)	105
80-proof	1 jigger (1½ ounces)	100
70-proof	1 jigger (1½ ounces)	85
Wines:		
Table wines (such as Chablis, claret, Rhine wine, and sauterne)	1 wine glass (about 3 ounces)	75
Dessert wines (such as muscatel, port, sherry, and Tokay)	1 wine glass (about 3 ounces)	125

Miscellaneous

		Number of calories
Bouillon cube	1 cube, ⅝ inch	5
Olives:		
Green	4 medium or 3 extra large or 2 giant	15
Ripe	3 small or 2 large	15
Pickles, cucumber:		
Dill	1 large, 1¾ inches in diameter by 4 inches long	15
Sweet	1 pickle, ¾ inch in diameter by 2¾ inches long	30
Popcorn, popped (with oil and salt added)	1 cup	65
Relishes and sauces:		
Chili sauce	1 tablespoon	20
Tomato catsup	1 tablespoon	15
Gravy	2 tablespoons	35
White sauce, medium (1 cup milk, 2 tablespoons fat, and 2 tablespoons flour)	½ cup	215
Cheese sauce (medium white sauce with 2 tablespoons cheese per cup)	½ cup	245

Appendix B

Weight Loss Chart

Starting weight: _____   Goal weight: _____

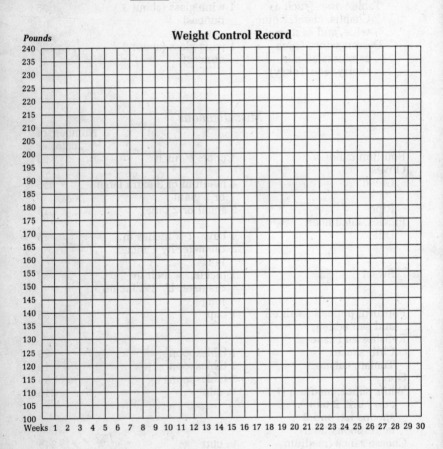

Pounds   **Weight Control Record**

Weeks 1 2 3 4 5 6 7 8 9 10 11 12 13 14 15 16 17 18 19 20 21 22 23 24 25 26 27 28 29 30